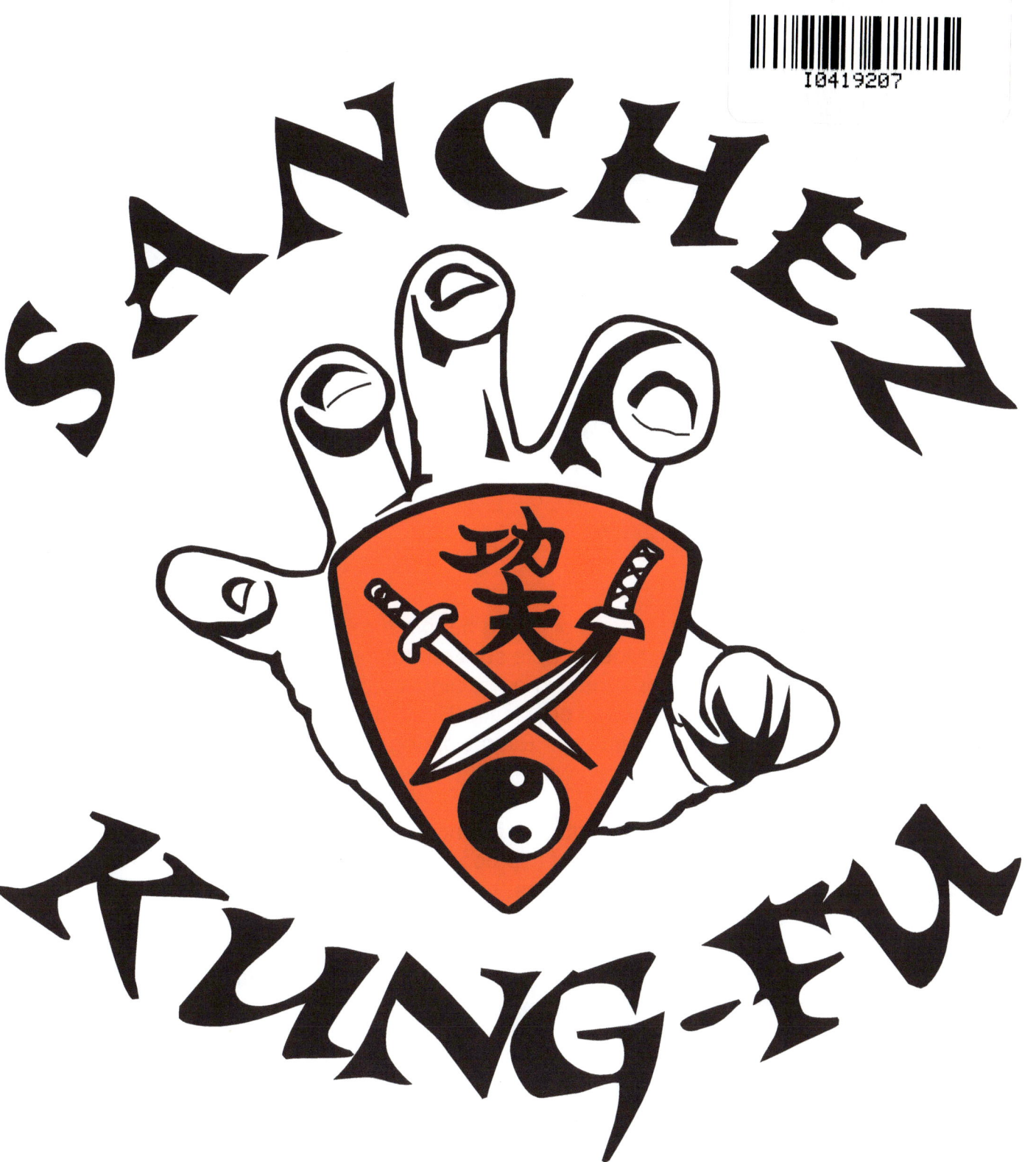

SANCHEZ

KUNG-FU

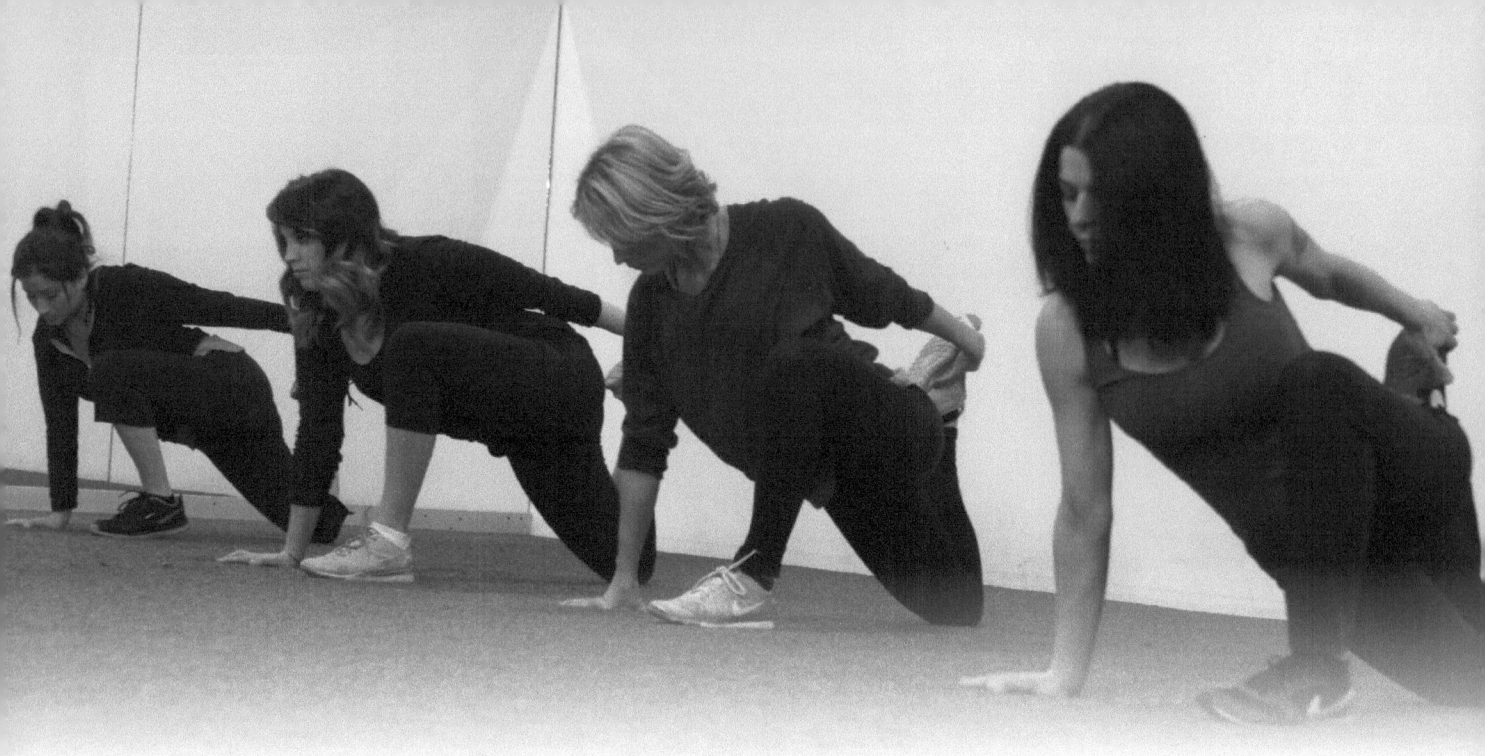

Forward

We put together this project with the idea of giving people a routine to stretch out the entire body in a simple, efficient manner. Most people start stretching after an injury and are doing some rehabilitation. We all know, or should know, maintaining some flexibility is important to the way our body functions, mentally and physically. Unfortunately, many feel stretching is not as important as the other aspects of fitness. Even working out has become less about being healthy and more about looking a certain way.

Physical fitness has three aspects: strength, endurance and flexibility. Unfortunately, flexibility is the most overlooked aspect. The focus of this book is to give people a stretching routine so they can work on the flexibility aspect of fitness.

Over three thousand years ago, Chinese Kung-Fu practitioners understood flexibility was important and implemented it in their teachings. As a result martial artists today are one of the most flexible athletic subsets of our population. In this booklet we will tap into the techniques that have made them so flexible.

Let us start by saying stretching is only one aspect of fitness. Stretching should be a part of every fitness program. Most people realize stretching is good to do, and most people know how to stretch a specific muscle or can at least figure it out when said muscle is tight. Our approach to this book is to put together a program on how to stretch out the entire body in a systematic approach with levels, so balance can be achieved.

Whether stretching to promote health and wellness or stretching before an event, a proper stretching routine is a workout in itself in which a great cleansing sweat may be achieved.

This booklet is set up as a guideline for stretching. Everyone is different, so everyone should expect to progress differently. Some stretches may never be fully achieved due to body type or previous injuries, etc. Do not worry about it. If one particular stretch is difficult for you, then this is the one on which you should spend a little extra time. Anderson (2006) suggests that flexibility, or the amount of flexibility one can achieve, is multi-factorial. Factors include: age, joint structure, gender, physical activity, fitness level and histology (anatomy of connective tissue).

Benefits of Stretching

What does stretching actually do for you? Stretching prepares a body for a workout, helps relax the body after a workout, helps eliminate waste products within the body, promotes injury prevention, and increases athletic performance if performed any time other than prior to the workout (Shrier 2004).

Do muscle, muscle tissue, tendons, joints, and ligaments all benefit from stretching? Yes, they do. When short, tight muscles are performing, stress is increased, causing micro tears, which leads to scar formation and further injury. Stretching will help decrease this common outcome. Stretching also promotes elimination of waste products and influx of nutrients to fuel these structures.

What are the medical benefits to stretching? There are many overall benefits. Some of these include:
- injury reduction and prevention
- mental stress reduction
- fall prevention in the elderly
- increase in athletic performance

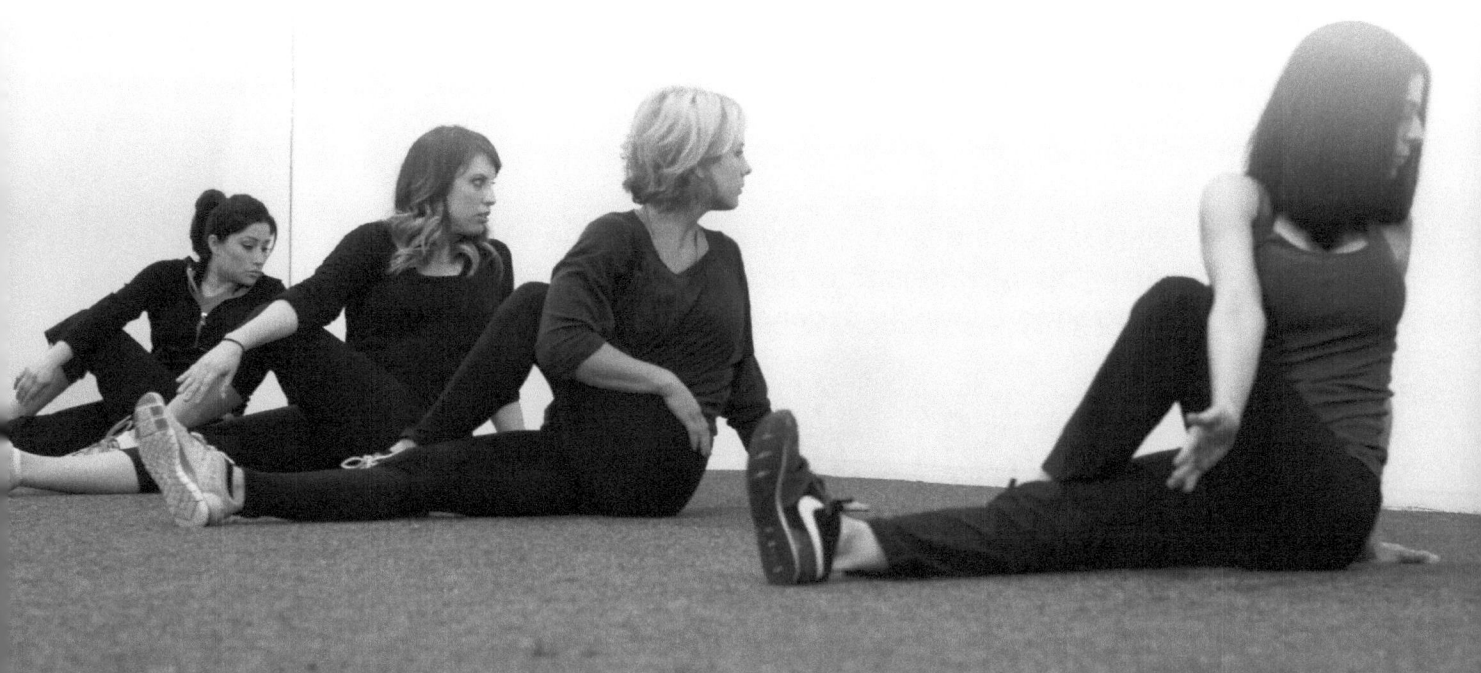

Does stretching align oneself? Short, tight, overactive muscles put asymmetric stress on the joints they cross over, therefore influencing the function of that joint. Stretching helps eliminate this problem and promote proper alignment. Having flexibility in one direction and not in another is known as asymmetry. A body with asymmetry is a body which is out of balance and likely to get injured.

Balance

Stretching has many benefits, one of which includes balance (equilibrium balance), depending on the type of stretching, if any, you've been taught. As we age, the need for balance is very important. We hear of the elderly doing fine until they have lost their balance and have fallen and broken a hip. Then they struggle afterwards to even walk in balance.

In the book we refer to balance in two methods.
- Stabilizing balance- equilibrium
- Equalizing strength throughout the body- having an equal balance of strength

Who Should Stretch?

All ages should stretch for different reasons. The elderly should stretch for fall prevention, middle age for maintenance of range of motion, and the young for athletic enhancement. Everyone should stretch regularly to prevent injury and improve range of motion. This booklet is not intended to diagnose or treat any physical ailments. If you are having any physical problems you should contact your doctor and have them direct your care.
Proper Technique

Is there a proper way to stretch? Current studies are showing that almost all stretching techniques are beneficial, including static, dynamic tension, PNF, ballistic, and active assisted. Some techniques require a trained partner because they can be a little more risky in terms of injury. Prior to stretching, doing some sort of warm-up is recommended. Warm muscles are going to be more effectively stretched. (Knight 2001) Self massage, foam rolling and/or stick work to prepare the muscles for stretching is the current trend, and this is perfectly acceptable as a warm-up.

How long does a person need to stretch? Studies show that 15-30 seconds is optimal time to stretch a muscle. Can you overstretch? Stretching to the point of injury is not recommended, and stretching a muscle more than 30 seconds is not time-efficient.

Proper Form

Is there proper form for stretching? Yes. In this book, we are targeting the proper stretching aspects. Proper form would include lengthening the muscle you are trying to stretch and lengthening the muscle enough to elicit the desired effect without causing injury. Breathe for relaxation of body and for muscle that is being stretched.

Concentrate on breathing with an inhale through the nose followed by an exhale through the mouth, in which one tries to relax the thoracic (chest) and diaphragmatic musculature (diaphragm). This in turn allows the body to relax more, which aides in stretching. Partner-assisted types of stretching require expertise from a trained professional because risk of injury is higher.

The key phrase that will be used multiple times throughout this book is PROPER FORM; without the knowledge of proper form, you will cheat yourself from the full purpose and benefits. An analogy would be like drying your hair with a paper towel. This would be viewed as improper form, whereas drying your hair with a cloth towel would be viewed as proper form. With a paper towel you will get a lot of water off, but you will also leave a lot of residue on your hair. A cloth towel, on the other hand, will get a much higher percentage of the water off/out leaving behind minimal residue.

That's how proper stretching versus improper stretching is. Instead of water residue being left behind that will eventually dry by itself, improper stretching form leaves behind lactic acid pockets as what we refer to as dead zones. This is where the blood is cheated from flowing freely in the stretch, which in turn results in no oxygen to the muscle and no flushing of the lactic acid residue – thus, like the paper towel. Where, on the other hand, proper stretching form allows a higher percentage of flushing to occur by maximizing stretching of muscle and tendons, opening the lines for blood to flow. This oxygenates and flushes the toxins to be replaced with a nutrient-enriched blood flow, leaving behind minimal residue, like the towel cloth.

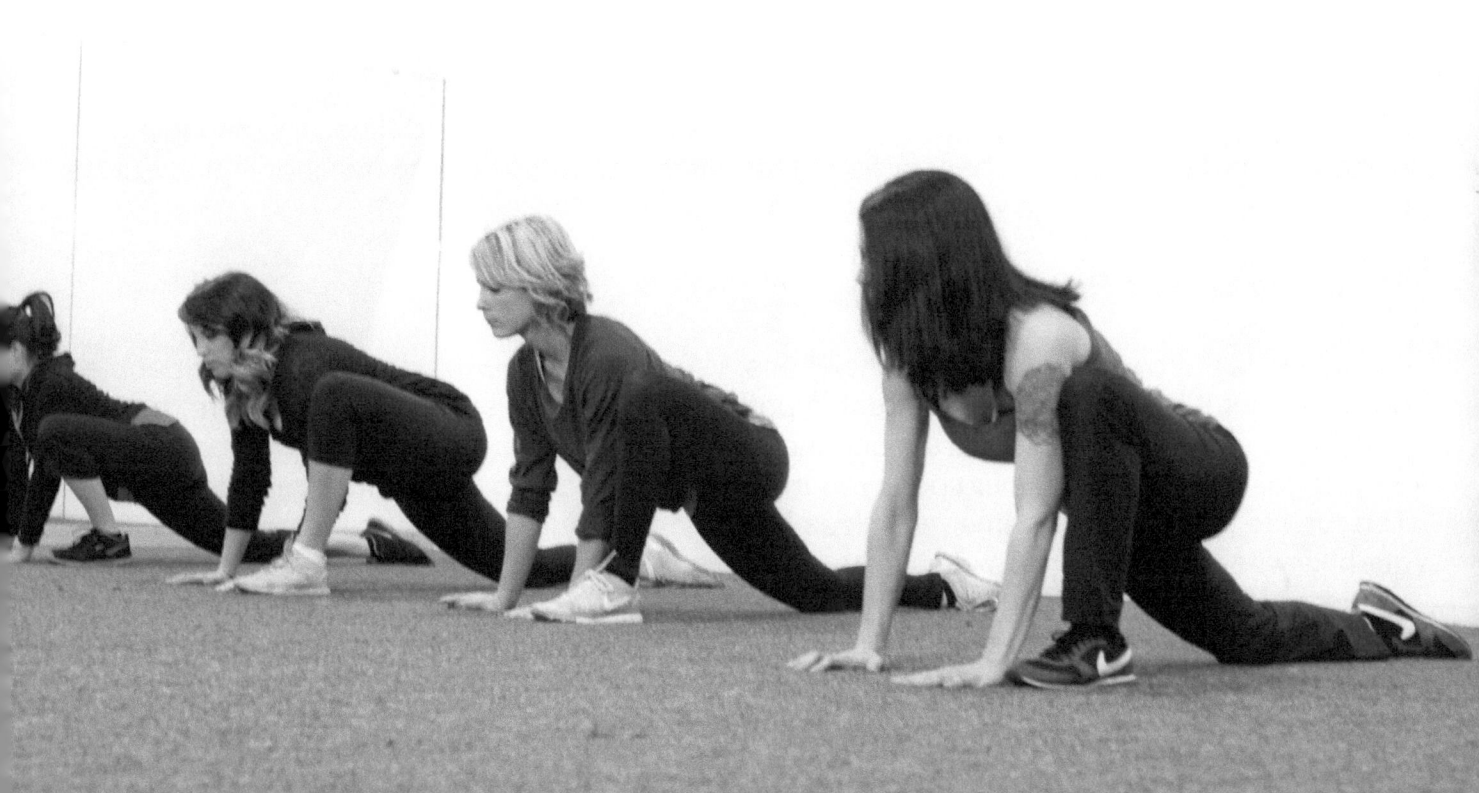

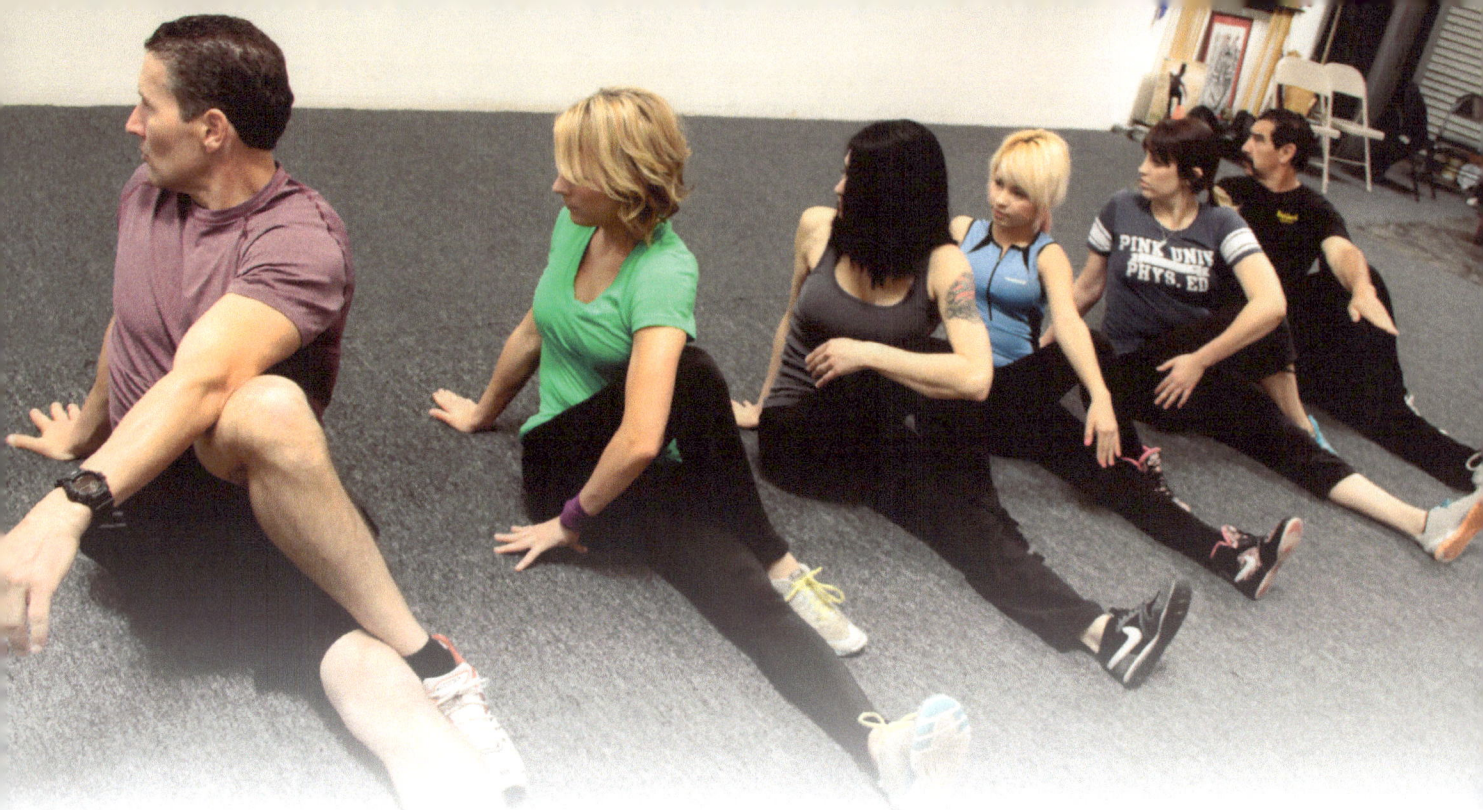

Eastern and Western philosophies differ in many ways.

Example
Eastern saying: "Long tendons, long life"
Western saying: "Don't forget to stretch" or "Be Sure to Stretch"

Stretching Western Views

Stretching is defined as: to lengthen, widen, or distend. Flexibility is defined as: capable of being bent or flexed, pliable, bent or flexed repeatedly without causing insult or injury. For the purposes of our booklet we will use stretching to achieve flexibility.

Stretching Eastern Philosophy

Stretching is the overlooked key to wholeness. When we talk about stretching, most people don't register it as a must-do or of great importance. In today's society, it's rush here, rush there! And in the athletic world it's much the same. A quick stretch, then a warm up, if any, and off you go. Depending on your sport, you may only be taught to stretch for five minutes or so. The rush to jump into the game minimizes or eliminates much importance to stretching. Consequently, when you see professional/elite athletes cramping and pulling muscles, it's mainly due to lack of oxygen to that particular muscle group. The lack of properly stretching increases your chances of cramping and/or pulling a muscle. You need to stretch to create blood flow and distribute oxygen throughout your body.

Followers of eastern philosophy of stretching in Chinese culture have been stretching for centuries and have made it part of everyday life, knowing the importance of keeping in harmony with the mind and the body. Even today in many Chinese communities you can still find the elderly in a local park or recreation center doing their early morning stretches, mainly the art of Tai Chi. Tai Chi is a series of organized movements that have multi benefits: breathing, balance, focus, stretch, strengthening of mental visualization, etc.

Stress!

With stretching as a means of stress relief, you will be amazed to feel how much stress you can simply stretch away! For most of us, stress or tension has become such an everyday part of our lives that we wear/carry it around with us and accept that it is just part of who we are. It becomes normal to us. News break! It's not normal to accept and give in to it. For one, it stagnates us; the Chinese call it lack of Chi (energy or flow). When the body is flowing correctly internally, it's like water in a stream - beautifully flowing, it seems to have no end. But when stress enters, it's like putting tiny sponges in the path or alongside the free-flowing stream. Parts of the water (flow) get pulled or locked into these sponges, which in turn does not allow the total amount of water to reach its destiny. When we internalize stress, it's like a little sponge that gets

Breathing

Breathing is the key to life - control your breathing, control your life. In other words, relaxed breathing is a relaxed person! Stress, anxiety, fear, smoking, hypertension etc. all create a change in breathing, which in turn creates an array of symptoms which include shortness of breath and panic. Then panic sets off a whole other cycle of symptoms. Stretching, or should we say one of the benefits of stretching, helps you control your breathing by calmly focusing on breathing pattern/technique during your stretch when taught by a qualified teacher. He or she will help you co-ordinate your stretching and breathing to work together in harmony, and harmony speaks for itself.

Placed somewhere in your body, ie. the mind, the hamstring, your chest, your stomach or at some point the entire body. When the entire body fills with these pockets of stress, we feel tired, lazy, lack of enthusiasm, etc. Then, if not addressed, it can escalate into an array of symptoms, body illnesses, or even depression. At that point, it's like an old semi-polluted water pond. It's water, but you can't really drink it until it goes through a filtering process. Stress can create that old pond feeling in you! But you can remedy that; you have a filtering process at your grasp! It's called stretching! Try it and take control; push out that stagnated (polluted) blood that represents stress. The pain you feel is the pain you'll heal! Drink plenty of water after every workout.

Anxiety/Worry

Anxiety is defined in its simplest term as an uneasiness of the mind. Anxiety can also be described as the lack of ability to decipher the outcome of something, be it present or future situations. There are many mental health professional recommendations for treating anxiety. One of the recommendations of treatment is meditation. What is meditation? It's a trained practice of visualization, be it visualizing a happy place, a calm place, positive affirmations or, in some practices, visualizing nothingness.

Great news! Stretching in itself can be a form of meditation. For example, while stretching when instructed correctly, you're taught to relax your breathing, align your body (correct form), and gently drop into your stretch. When you reach the point of tension, take about 10 seconds minimum to relax at that point; then take a deep breath, inhale through the nose and, during your exhale through the mouth, gently drop a bit deeper into the stretch. Keep proper form at all times. If you stretch your entire body, it becomes a multi-meditation process, thus creating an exhilarating sense of calmness and relaxation. Once relaxed, you can understand that anxiety/worry is a choice, either conscious or subconscious. Stretching may be used as a method of just letting go. Choose to be happy, act happy and guess what? Knowledge is power!

STRETCHING BASICS

BREATHE · STRETCH · RELAX

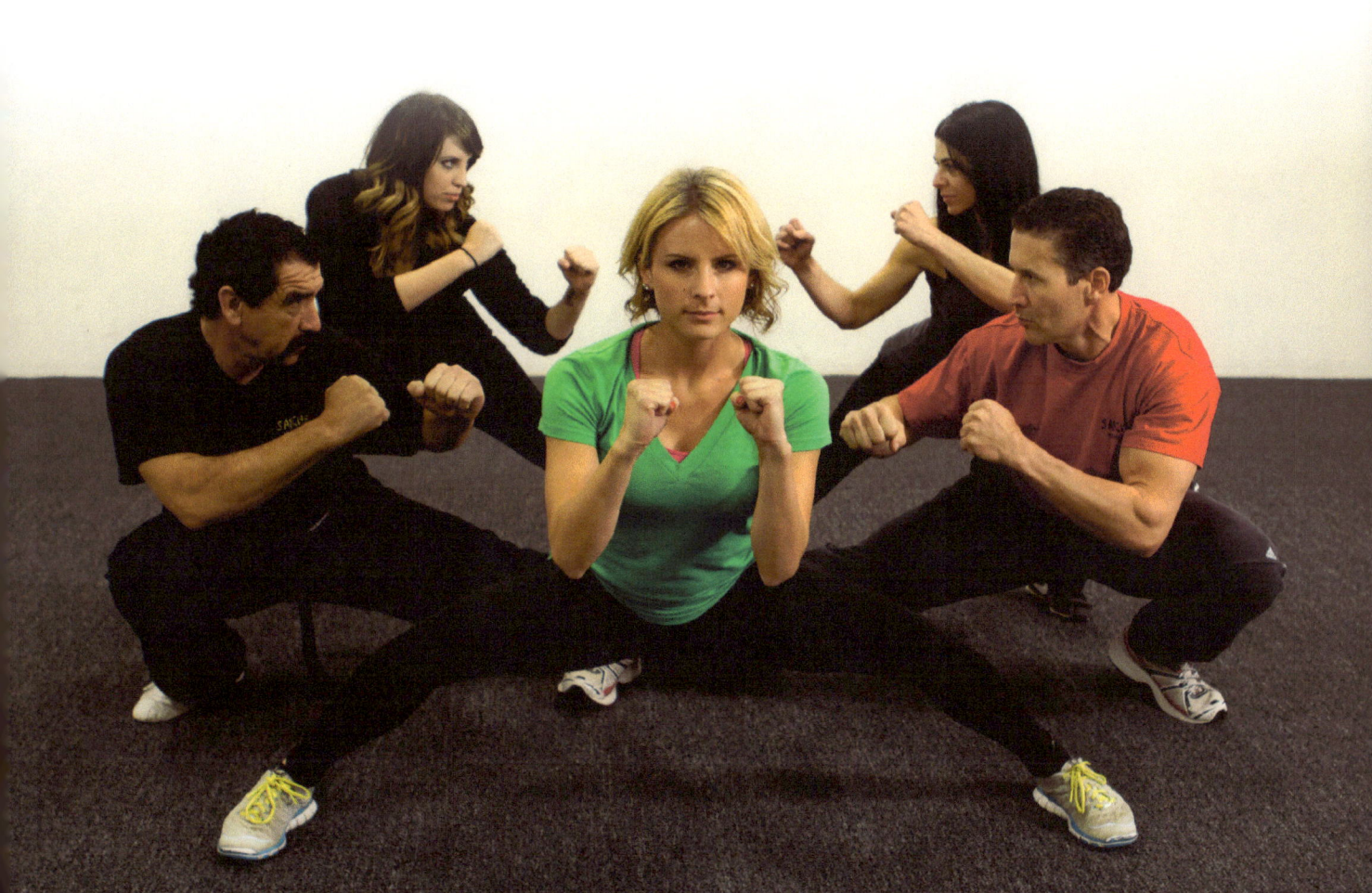

Groin/Hamstring Stretch

- From the standing position and move legs apart, left foot to 9 o'clock, right foot to 3 o'clock.
- Place hands palm down with fingers touching, on the ground in front of you.
- Inhale, and then, as you exhale, drop the upper body down and bend both elbows outwards until forearms are on the ground.
- Keep the back as straight as possible, for proper form.

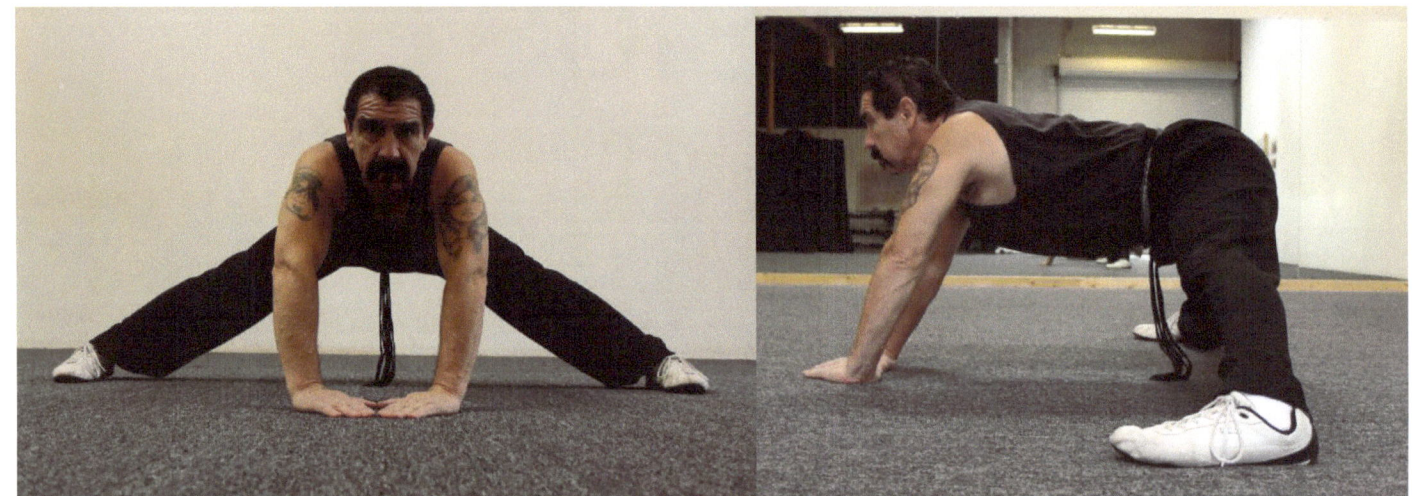

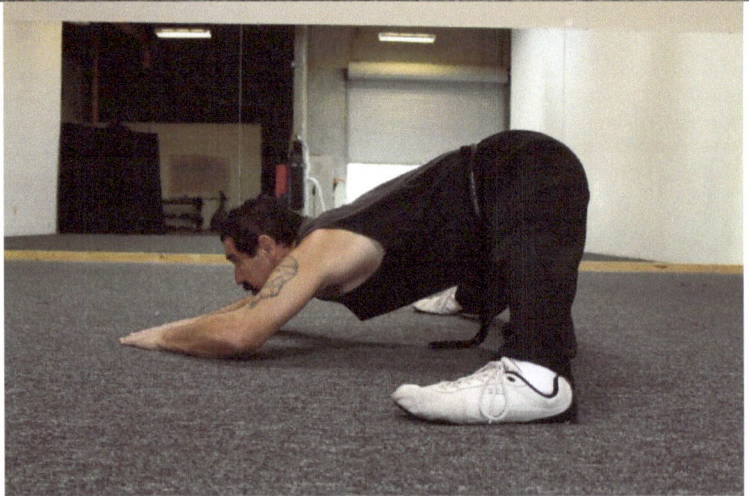

From the standing position. Move the legs apart by doing the side splits, left foot to 9 o'clock, right foot to 3 o'clock.

Put your hands on the ground in front of you, with thumbs and index fingers touching, and then inhale.

As you exhale, body down, and bend both elbows outward until forearms are flush to the ground. If possible, to increase the stretch, inhale and as you exhale, push the body back, and lift hips upward toward ceiling. Keep the back as straight as possible for proper form.

Groin Stretch

- Assume the all-fours position and place the right leg straight out to 3 o'clock, as far as possible.
- Inhale and then as you exhale, roll the right leg/glute down and back. This will stretch the hamstring and groin area.
- Inhale, and then, as you exhale, drop the chest straight down, keeping the back straight while trying to place the forearms on the ground.
- Repeat for other side.

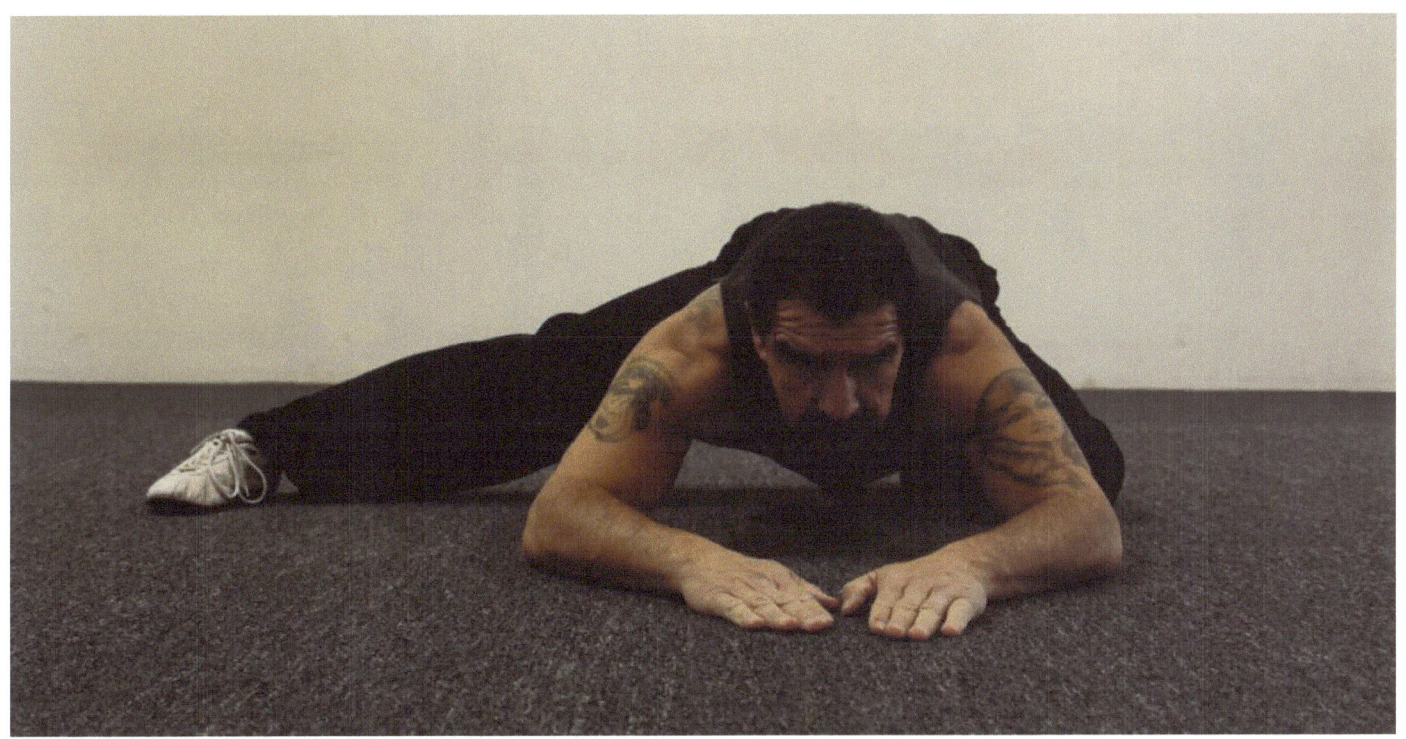

Assume the all fours position. Place the left knee in the nine o'clock position. Place the right leg clear out in the 3 o'clock position. Maximize the stretch by extending the left knee further towards the 9 o'clock position. Next, inhale, and then, as you exhale, roll the right leg/glute down and back; this will stretch the hamstring and groin area.

Again, to maximize the stretch, inhale deeply, and then, as you exhale drop the chest straight down, keeping the back straight. It's best, for the flexibility, to place the forearms on the ground.

Hamstring Stretch Side Position

- Assume the kneeling position, and place the right leg out towards 3 o'clock.
- Point the toes up and back.
- Place the left hand on the left waist/hip.
- Inhale, and then, as you exhale, use the right hand to grab the right foot, if possible. Otherwise, grab the shin or the middle of the thigh.
- Inhale, and then, as you exhale, pull the upper body down toward 2 o'clock while bending the elbow towards the ceiling.
- Repeat through a couple of breathing cycles.
- Repeat exercise on the other side.

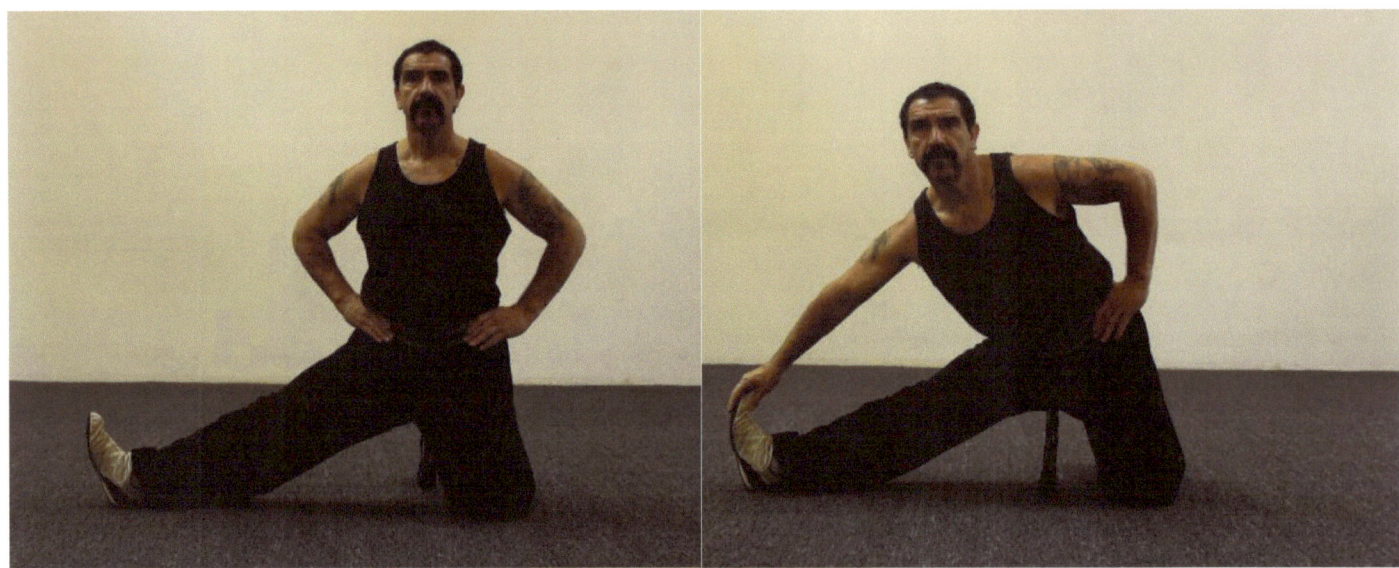

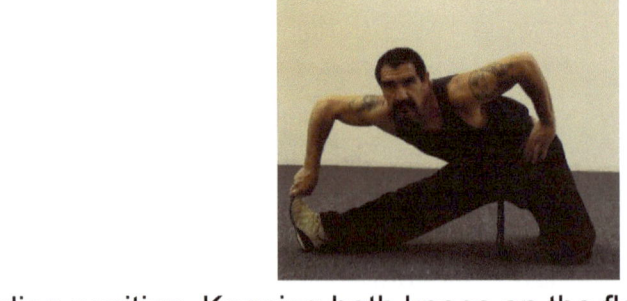

Assume the kneeling position. Keeping both knees on the floor in a bent knee position, move the right leg out to 3 o'clock. Point the toes up and back. This is a simple angle stretch. Put the left hand on the left waist/hip. Inhale, and then as you exhale, use the right hand to grab the right foot. If not possible, grab the shin or middle of the thigh. To intensify the stretch, pull the toe back.

Next, inhale, and then, as you exhale, move the upper body down toward 2 o'clock while bending the elbow toward the ceiling.

Note: Keep the back as straight as possible. If hard on the knees, use a knee pad or pillow.

Hamstring Stretch Forward Position

- Assume the kneeling position, place the hands on the hips and extend the right leg out in front of you.
- Heel down, place midline of the right leg in line with the center of the body, and place the toes up and back toward right knee.
- Inhale, and then, as you exhale, while keeping a straight back, lean the upper body forward. At the same time grab the thigh.
- Inhale again, and, as you exhale, lean upper body forward, and bend elbows outward. While lowering the chest slowly downward towards the right thigh, keep the back straight.
- As flexibility increases, repeat above steps, grabbing lower on the leg. Ultimately, you should be able to grab the foot.

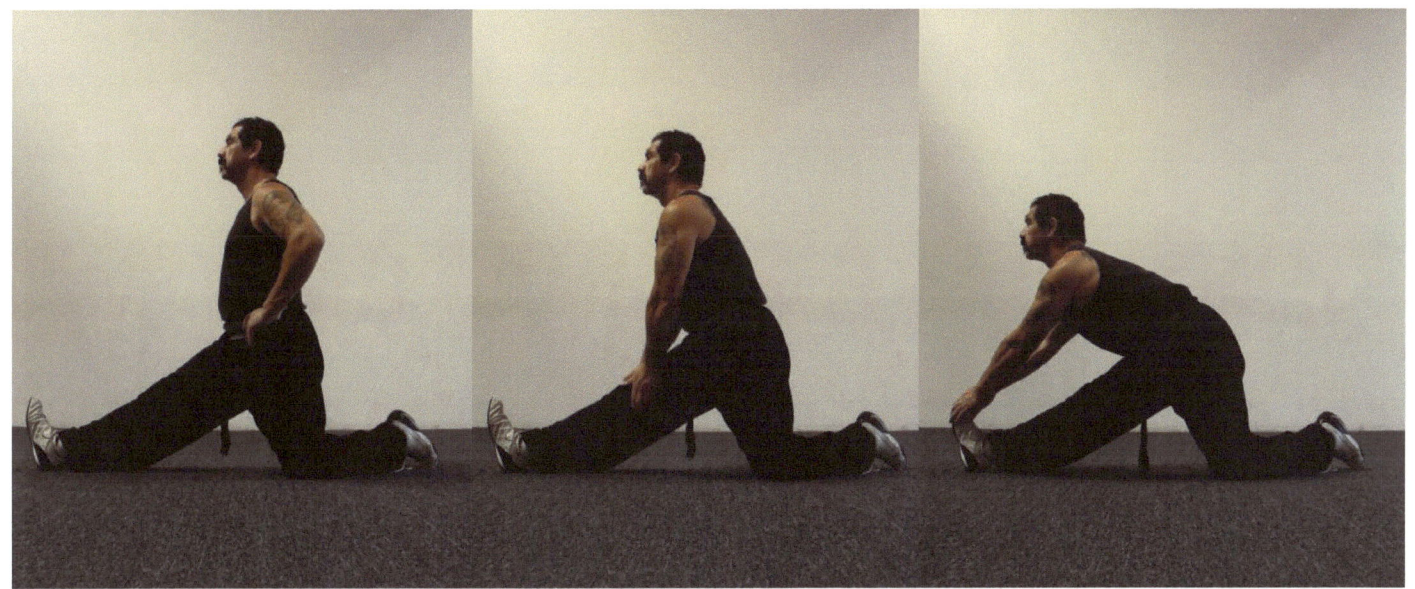

Assume the kneeling position, and place the hands on the hips. Extend the right leg out in front of you, with the heel down and toes pointed up and back toward right knee. If possible and for best results, place the extended leg at an angle even with the center of the chest. Keeping the back straight, inhale, and, as you exhale, lean the upper body forward. At the same time, place both hands on the thigh, inside and outside.

Next, inhale again; then, as you exhale, lean the upper body forward, and bend elbows outward. Keep the back straight, and slowly lower the chest downward towards the right thigh. As flexibility improves, repeat the above movements, and attempt to place the hands further down on the thigh, then down to shin area, and then, ultimately, grab the foot.

Straight Arm Tricep Stretch

- Assume the kneeling (or standing) position, and place right arm across chest, towards the left shoulder.
- Using the left hand, grab just above the right elbow.
- Lift the right arm toward the neck.
- Lean the right shoulder out to the right side.
- Repeat exercise on other side.

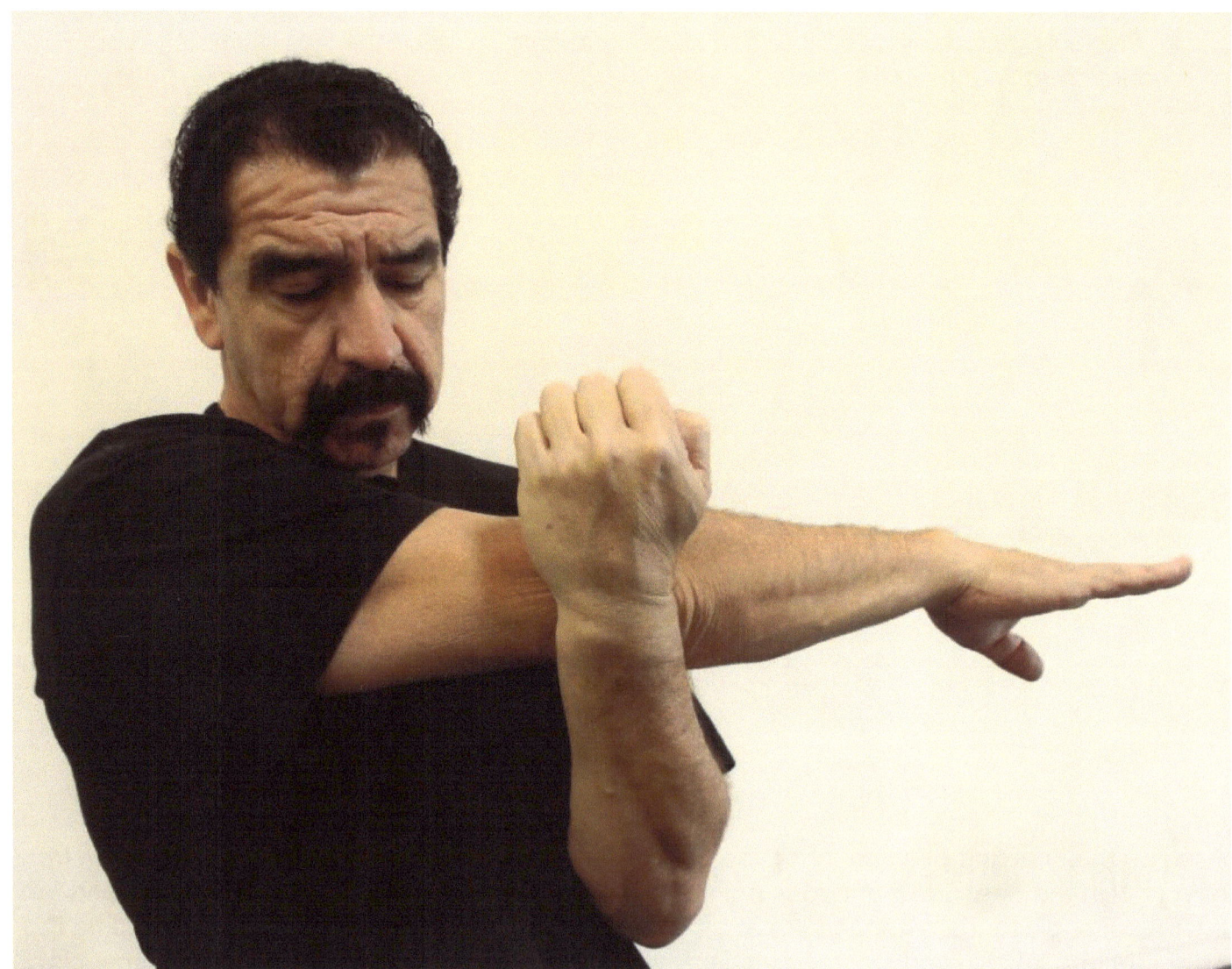

Assume the kneeling or standing position. Place the right arm across the chest, towards the left shoulder. Using the left hand, grab at the base of the triceps just above the elbow. Lift the right arm toward the neck. A deeper stretch is possible by leaning the right shoulder out to the right side.

Note: The pulling hand, just above the elbow, may utilize either the fist or palm.

Bent Arm Tricep Stretch

- Assume the kneeling or standing position. Place right arm across the chest.
- Right hand wraps around the left hand side of the neck.
- Place left palm at the right arm just above the elbow.
- Pull right arm toward left shoulder.
- Lean the right shoulder away to intensify the stretch.
- Repeat exercise on the other side.

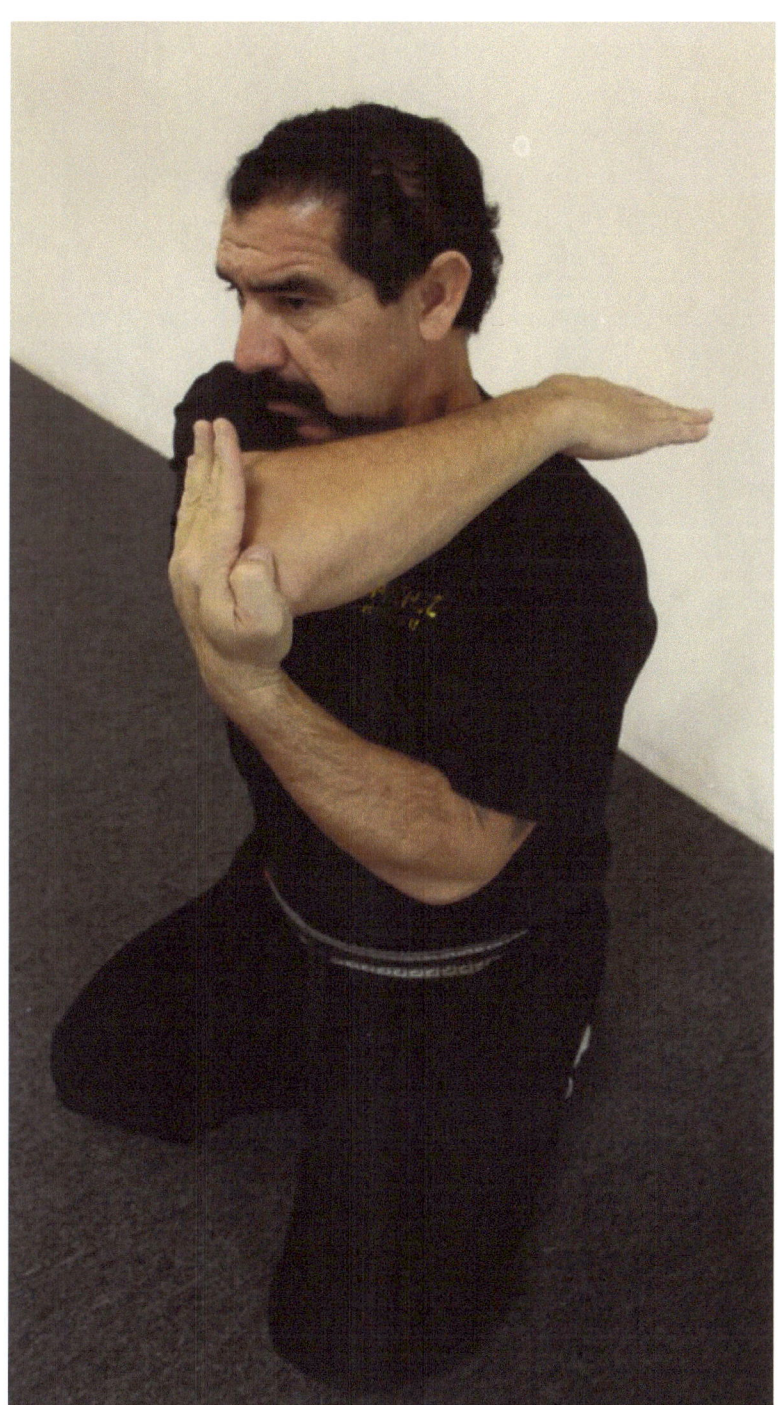

Assume the kneeling or standing position. This stretch is similar to the straight arm stretch. Place the right arm across the chest. Wrap the right hand around the left side of the neck, like choking yourself. Place the left palm at the right elbow base. Pull toward the left shoulder, and lean the right shoulder away to intensify the stretch. Repeat exercise with the other arm.

Note: The pulling hand may use either the fist or the palm.

Bicep Stretch

- Assume the kneeling or seated position.
- Place the right arm, palm down, with the fingers pointed back towards the right leg.
- Make the left hand into a fist and place it underneath the chest at the tricep.
- Inhale, and then, as you exhale, push the palm down and try to lift the fingers off the ground. There should be a feeling of stretching the bicep.
- The key is in the fingers, pulling them back and upwards.
- Repeat exercise for the other arm.

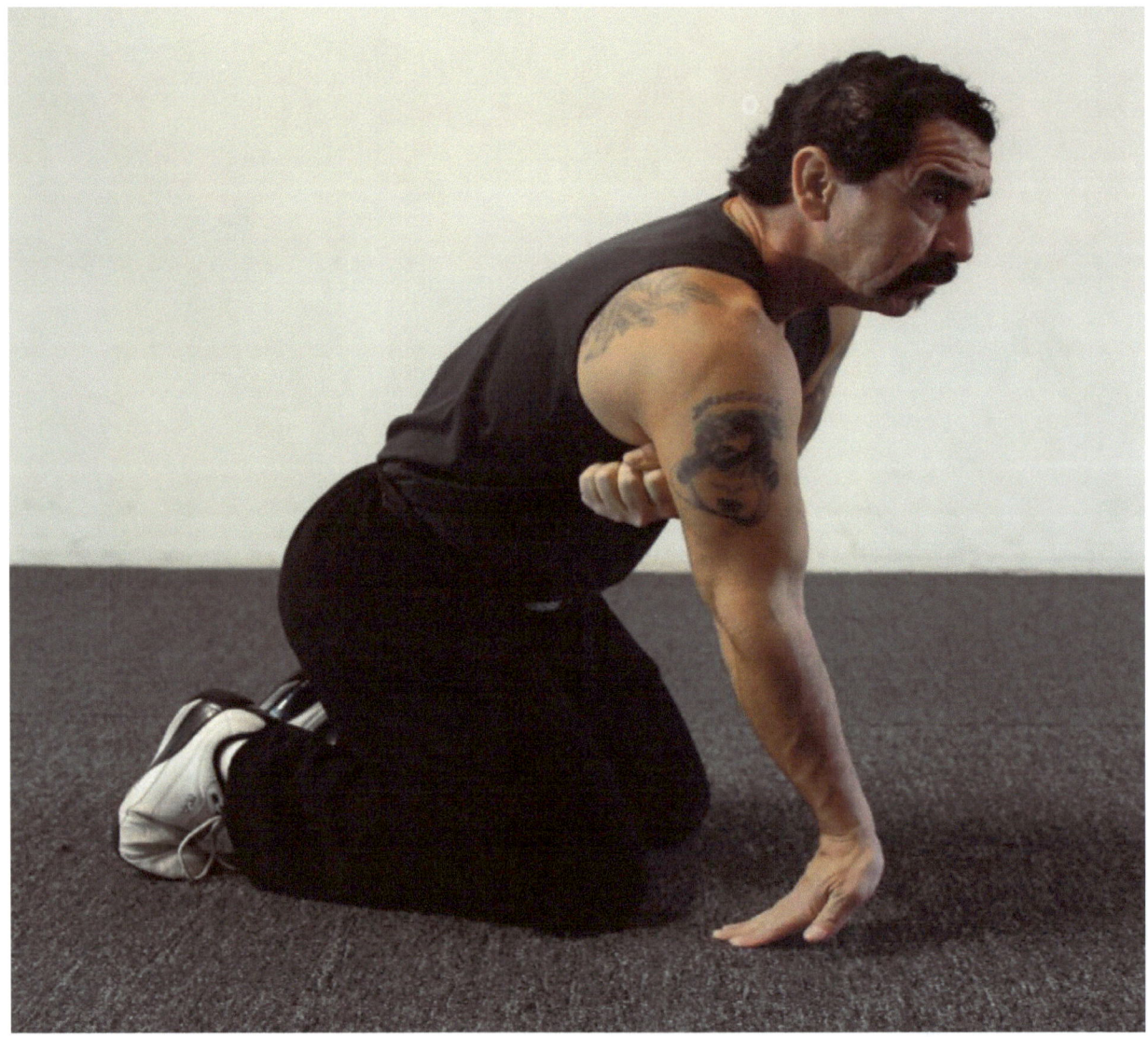

Assume the kneeling or seated position. Using the right arm, point the palm down with the fingers pointed back towards the right leg. Make the left hand into a fist, and place it underneath the chest at the tricep. Inhale and then as you exhale, push the palm down, and try to lift fingers off the ground. You should feel a stretching of the bicep. The key is in the fingers, pulling them back and upwards. Repeat exercise, using the other arm.

Back of the Forearm Stretch

- Assume the kneeling position, and place back side of the index finger on the ground.
- Straighten elbows.
- Drop the weight of the upper body downward, until you feel a stretch on the outer part of the forearm and slightly on the wrist.

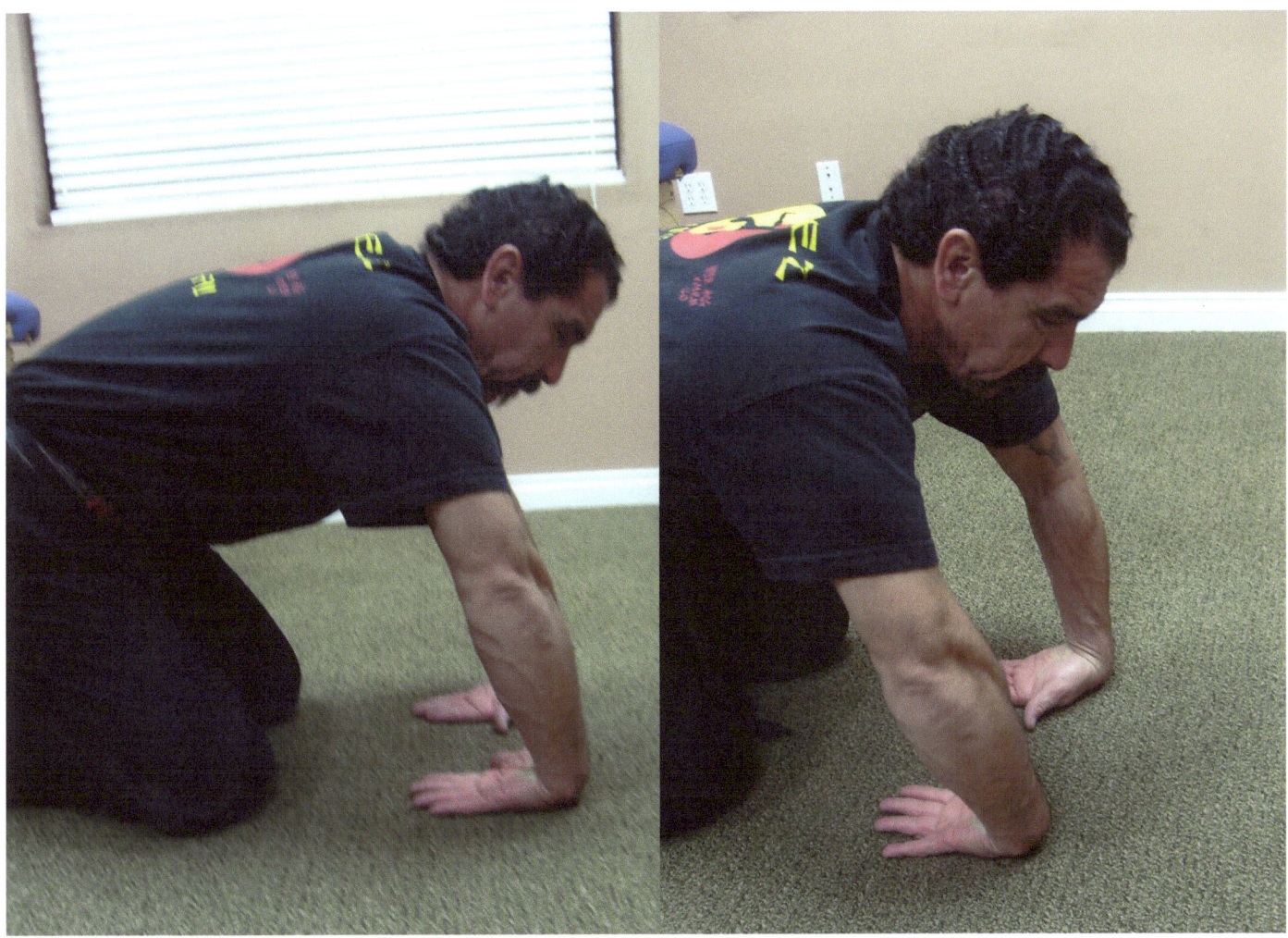

Assume the kneeling position. This stretch is for the outside portion of the wrist and forearm. Place both hands in front, with only the index finger knuckle touching the ground. Gage the stretch by dropping the weight of the upper body downward until you feel a stretch on the outer part of the forearm and slightly on the wrist. The application is the large index knuckle only.

Chest / Shoulder Stretch

- Assume the all-fours position, and extend the right arm to the 3 o'clock position with the palm down.
- Inhale, and then, as you exhale, drop the right shoulder down and to the left.
- Repeat through a couple of breathing cycles.
- Repeat exercise on the other side.

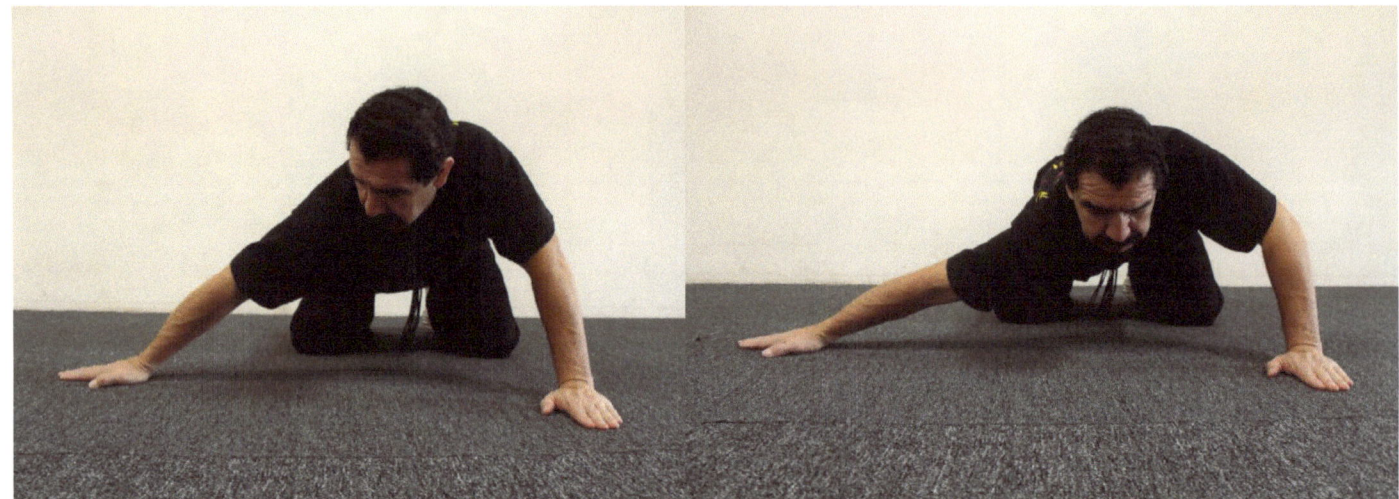

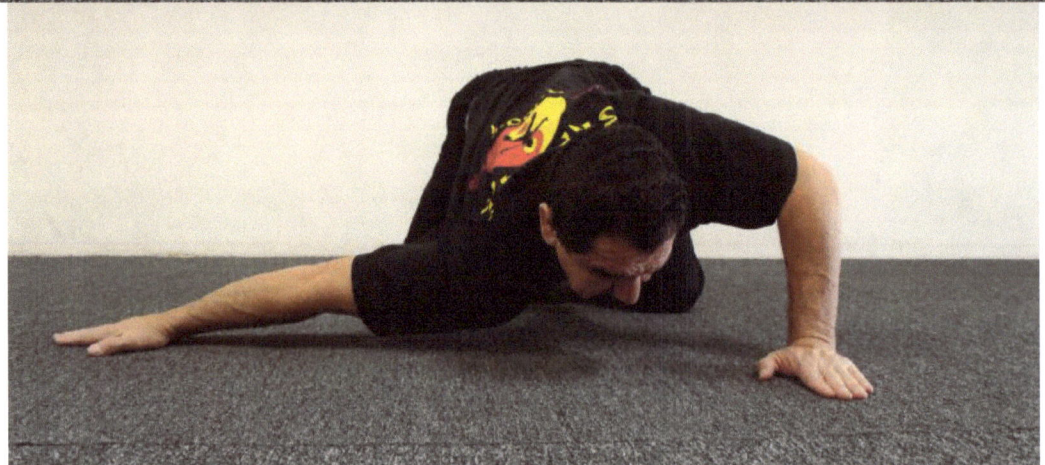

Assume the all-fours position. Place the right hand in the 3 o'clock position, and extend it out with the palm down. Inhale and then as you exhale, drop the right shoulder down and to the left. Try to bring the shoulder to the other hand without moving the right hand. Repeat exercise using the other arm.

Tricep / Back of Shoulder Stretch

- Assume the all-fours position, and place the left hand at the 12 o'clock position.
- Place the right arm, with the palm up, behind the left arm.
- Inhale, and then, as you exhale, drop the right shoulder down slowly and away from hands.
- Repeat exercise on the other side.

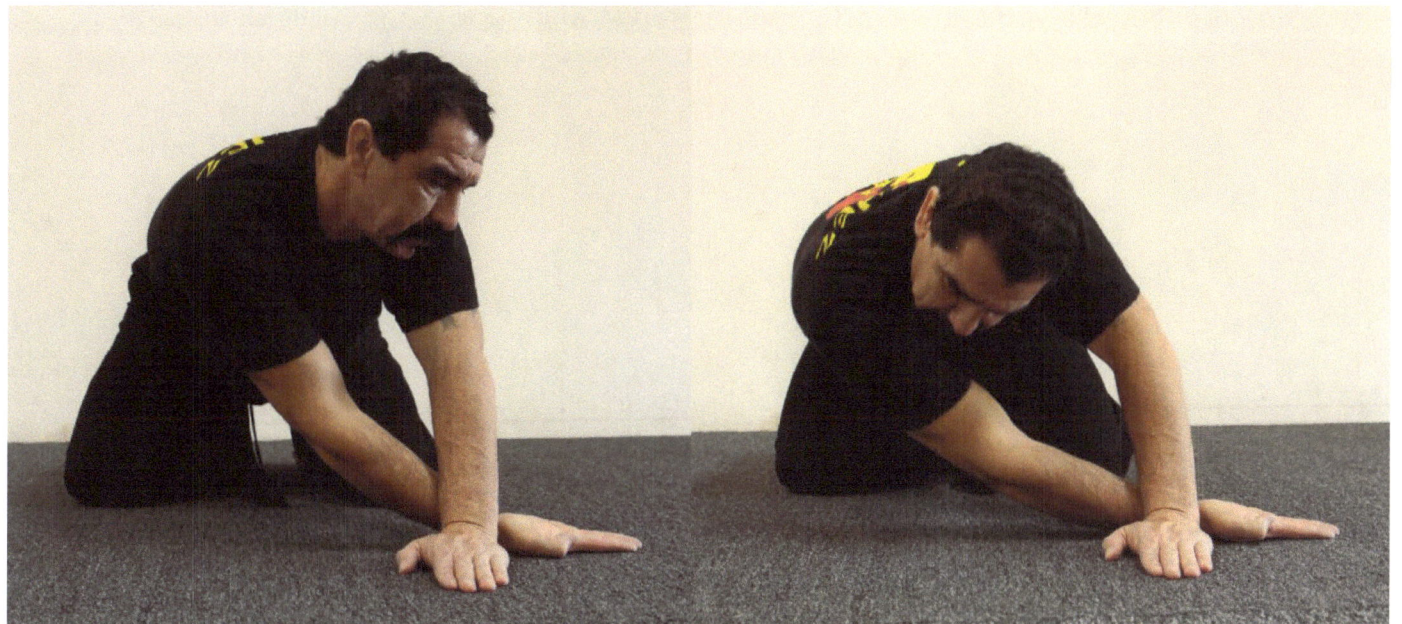

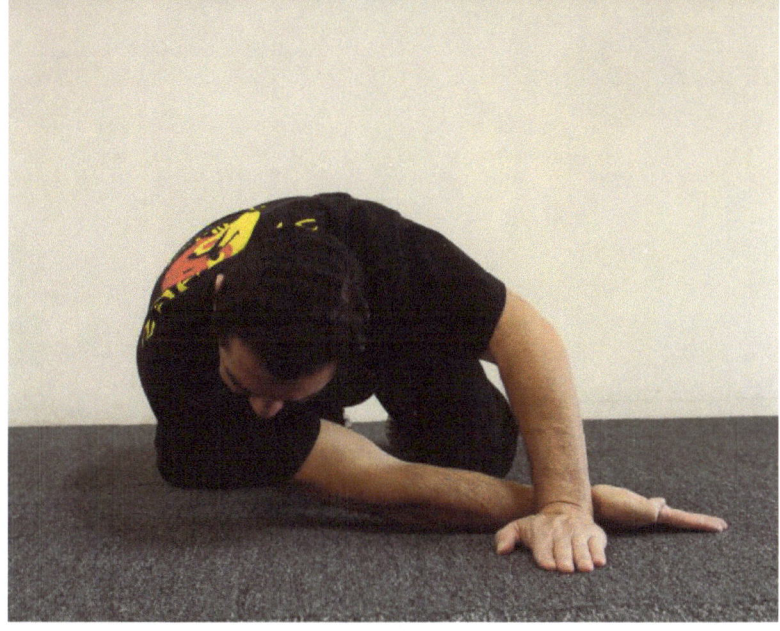

Assume the all-fours position, and place the left hand at the 12 o'clock position. Place the right arm, with the palm up, behind the left arm. Inhale and then as you exhale, drop the right shoulder down slowly and away from the hands. Repeat exercise on the other side.

Note: Do not let hands move while slowly dropping the shoulder.

3-Part Quadricep Stretch

Position 1

- Assume the push-up position, and place the right leg forward with the bottom of the foot flat on the floor.
- Move the left leg straight back, to the 6 o'clock position.
- Place the hips square.
- Inhale, and then, as you exhale, drop that left hip straight down and roll it forward.

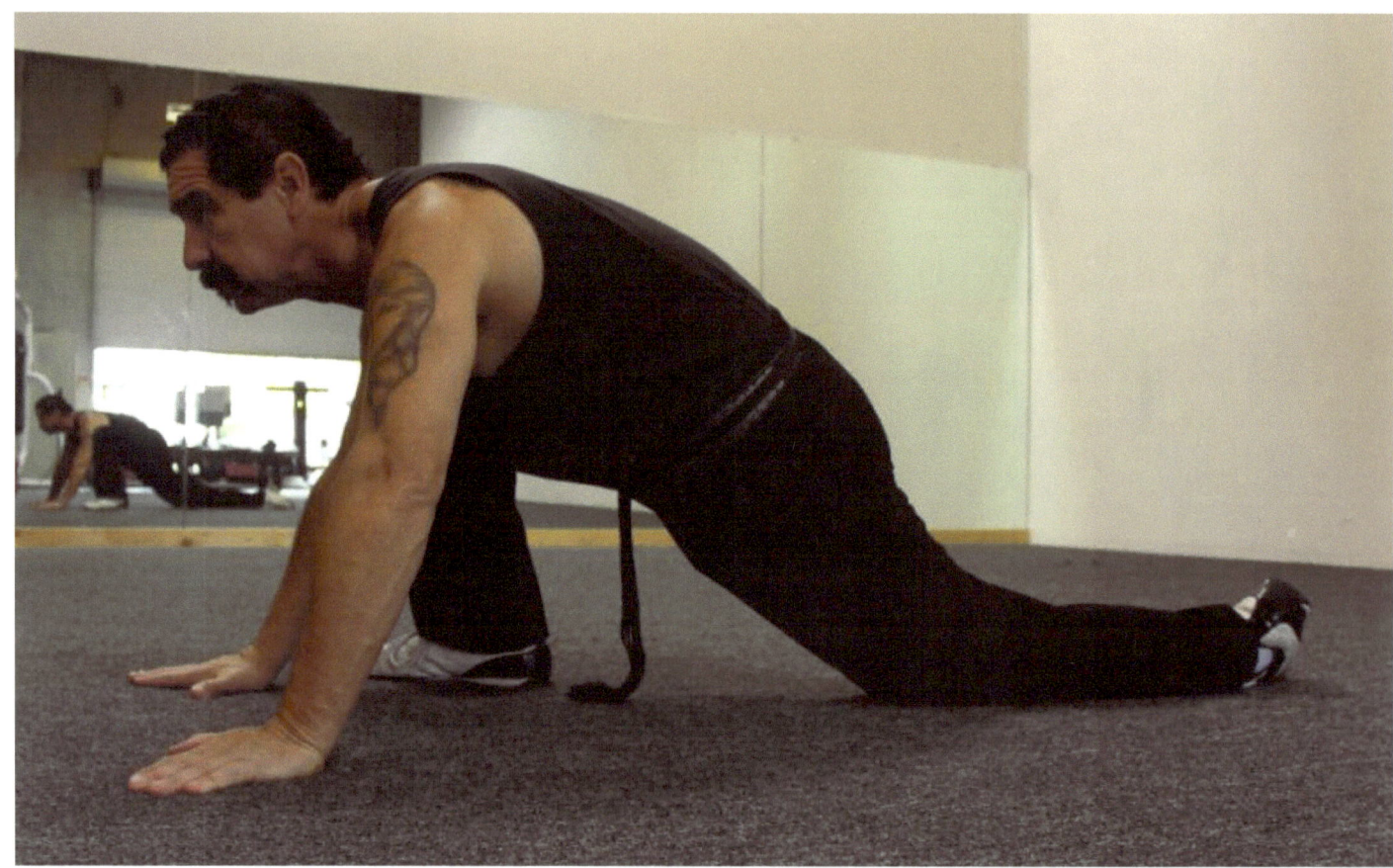

Assume the push-up position, and bring the right leg forward with the bottom of the foot flat on the floor. Place the right arm to the inside of the right knee to support it. Place the left leg straight back, to the 6 o'clock position, with the foot pointing to the 5 o'clock position. The hips should be square.

Inhale and then as you exhale, drop that left hip straight down and roll it forward. Don't let the knee move while rolling the hip bone forward.

3-Part Quadricep Stretch

Position 2
- Reach back with the right hand, and grab the left foot.
- Bending the left knee, pull the left foot to the left glute.
- Lower the left hip down toward the ground.
- Inhale, and then, as you exhale, lower it more and roll the hip bone forward.

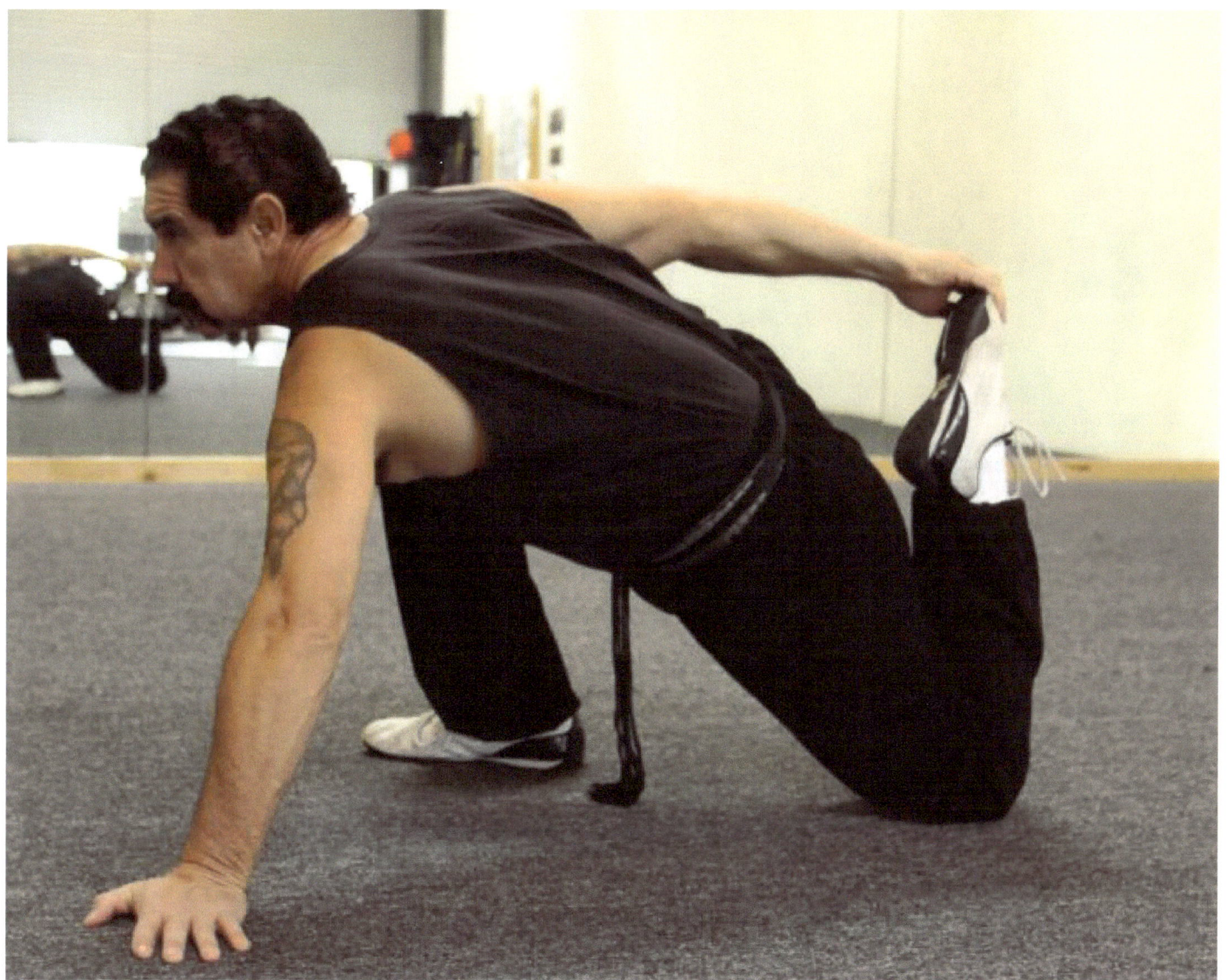

Place your right hand behind the back, bend the left leg up to grab the left foot (or the ankle or pant leg) with the right hand. Lower the left hip down toward the ground until you feel the tension.

Inhale, and then, you exhale, lower it more and roll the hip bone forward. The goal is to be able to grab the foot.

3-Part Quadricep Stretch

Position 3
- Switch the hand that is holding the foot.
- Inhale, and then, as you exhale, drop and rotate that left hip bone down and forward.

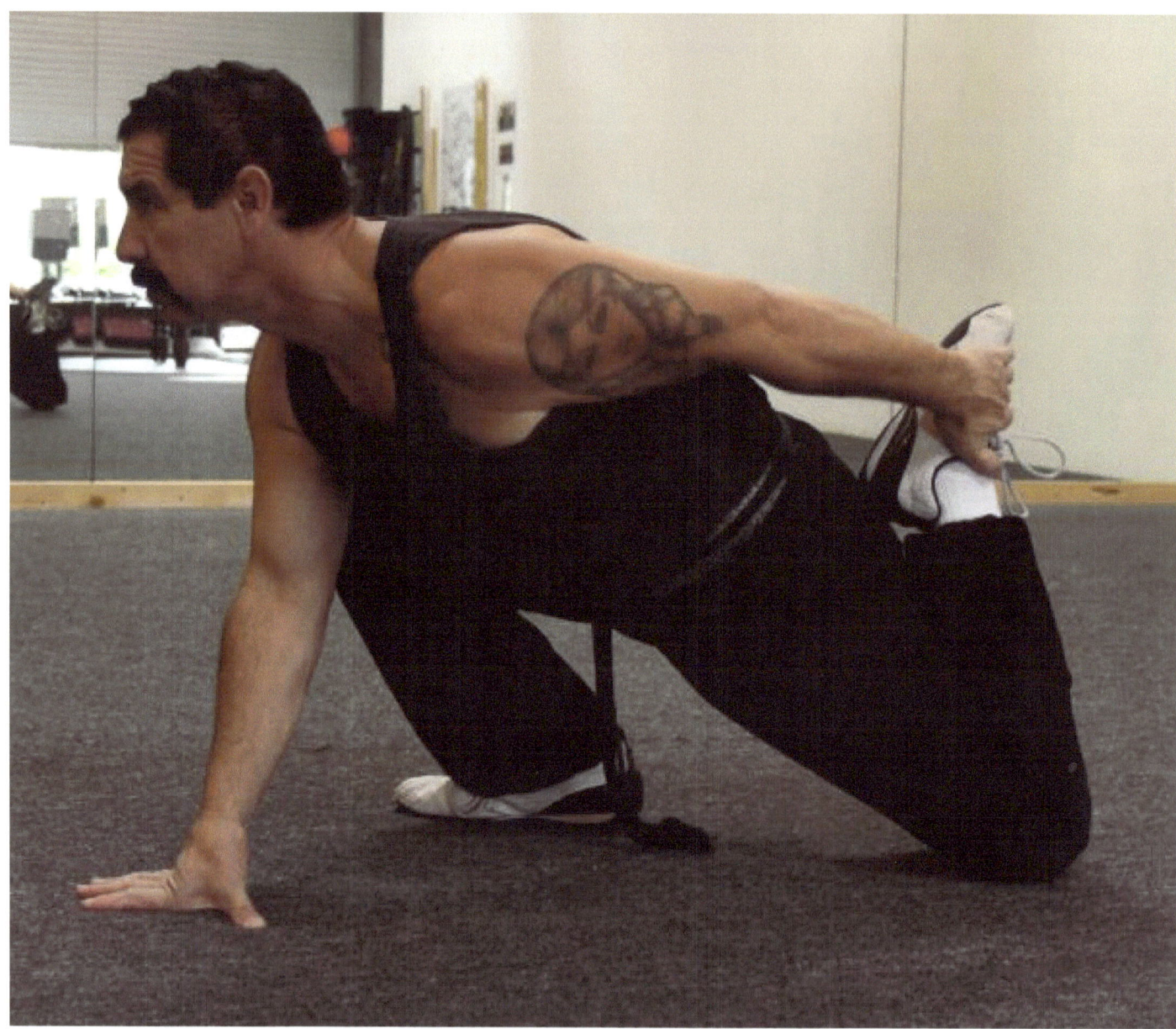

Switch hands. Put the right hand back inside the right knee, or slightly in front is acceptable. Use the left hand to grab the left foot. This will keep yourself perfectly square. Tension should be felt, immediately upon grabbing the left foot. Inhale and then as you exhale, drop and rotate that left hip bone down and forward.

Note: The ultimate goal is to be able to grab the foot. If this is not possible, grab the pants leg.

Hip Flexor Stretch

- Assume the all-fours position with the hands in a push up mode.
- Bring the left knee forward, and place the foot flat on the ground.
- Extend the right leg to the left, crossing it behind the left foot.
- Inhale, and then, as you exhale, slowly lower that right hip bone straight down.
- Repeat exercise on the other side.

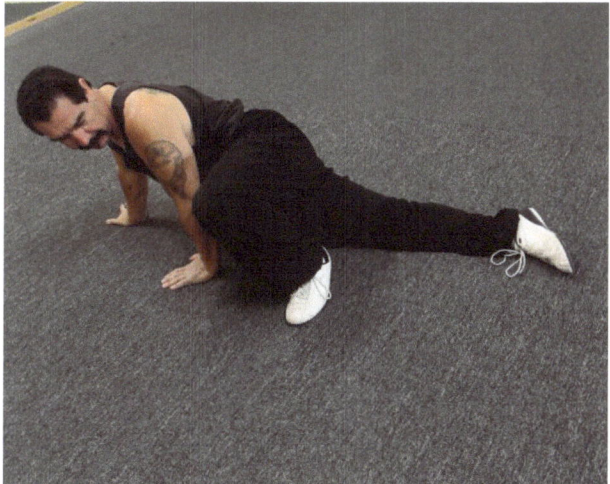

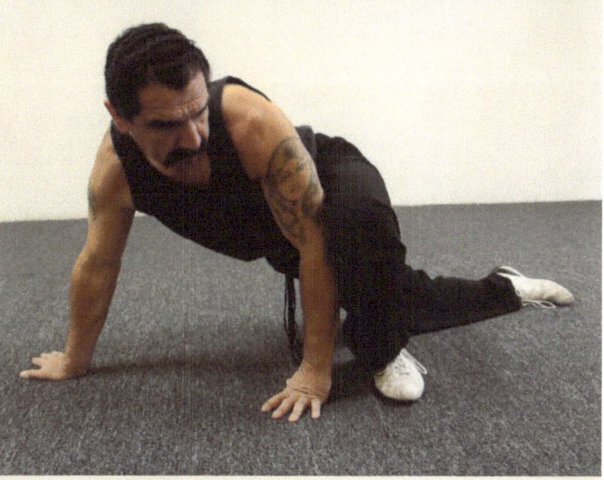

Assume the all-fours position with the hands in a push-up mode. Move the left knee up and bend it while kneeling on the right knee. Place hands out in front at 12 o'clock, and cross the right leg to the left, crossing behind the left foot. The right leg will have a little angle on it. Keep the right hip elevated. Roll that leg slightly forward in order to create the center of the thigh even with the ground and the hip bone pointing straight down to the ground.

Inhale and then as you exhale, slowly lower that right hip bone straight down, and that will create the hip flexor stretch. Be sure that bent knee is right up against the arm in order to stabilize the knee.

Repeat exercise on the other side.

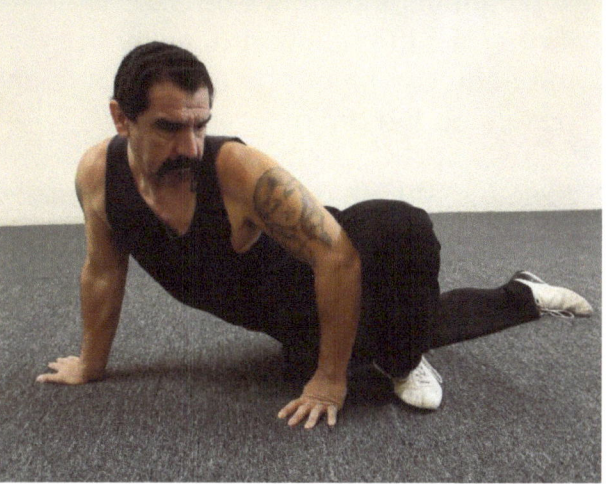

Groin Stretch

- Assume the all-fours position, and place the bottom of the feet together behind you.
- Inhale, and then, as you exhale, slowly lower the hips toward the ground.
- Attempt to lower the buttocks to the ground while moving the body closer to the arms.

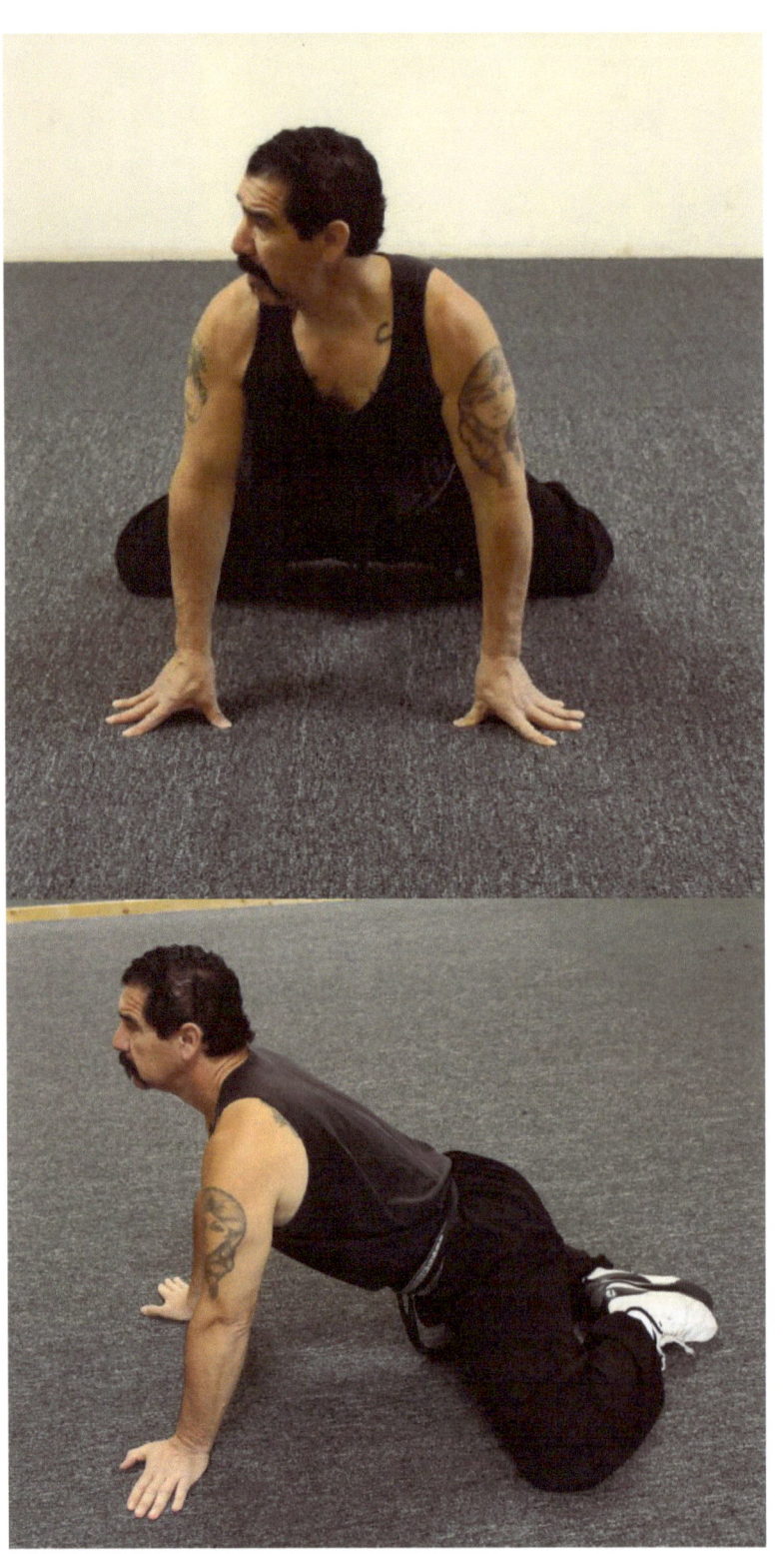

Assume the all-fours position. Spread the knees, left knee to 9 o'clock and right knee to 3 o'clock. Join the bottom of the feet together behind. There are two variations on this exercise: The further out the hands are, away from the body, the higher up that this stretch occurs on the groin.

Breathe in deeply, and as you exhale, slowly lower the hips toward the ground. To obtain the full benefit of this stretch, attempt to lower the belly/buttocks to the ground while moving the arms closer to the body.

3-Part Outer Thigh and Glute Stretch

Position 1
- Assume the sitting position. Adjust position, to sit on the outer part of the right leg, with the knees bent.
- Place the right knee to point at 1 o'clock and the right foot to point at 9 o'clock.
- Place the right hand out in front of the right knee. This will introduce you to the stretch.

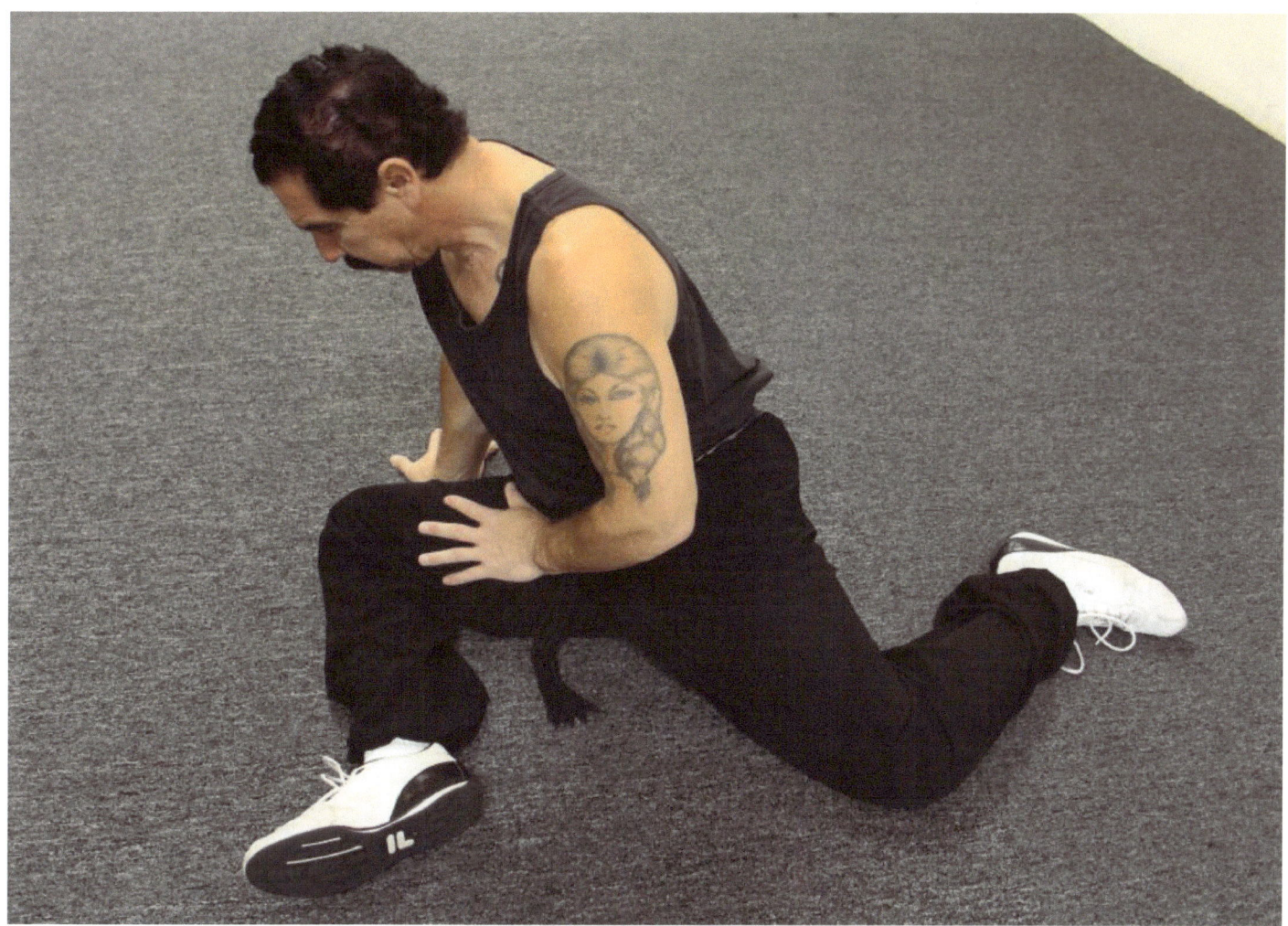

Assume the sitting position. For the outer part of the lead leg stretch, sit on the outer part of the right leg. The right calf is going to be right in front of you. The knee will be at 1 o'clock, and the foot will be somewhere near 9 o'clock. You may adjust where you want to stretch, by moving the foot away or towards the body. Place the left leg behind you and bent in a comfortable position.

This stretch is for the front leg. Place the right hand out in front and away from the right knee. Take it straight out. This will introduce you to the stretch.

3-Part Outer Thigh and Glute Stretch

Position 2

- From position one, inhale, and then, as you exhale, move the right hand way out in front of the bent knee as shown above. Light tension should be felt on right leg.

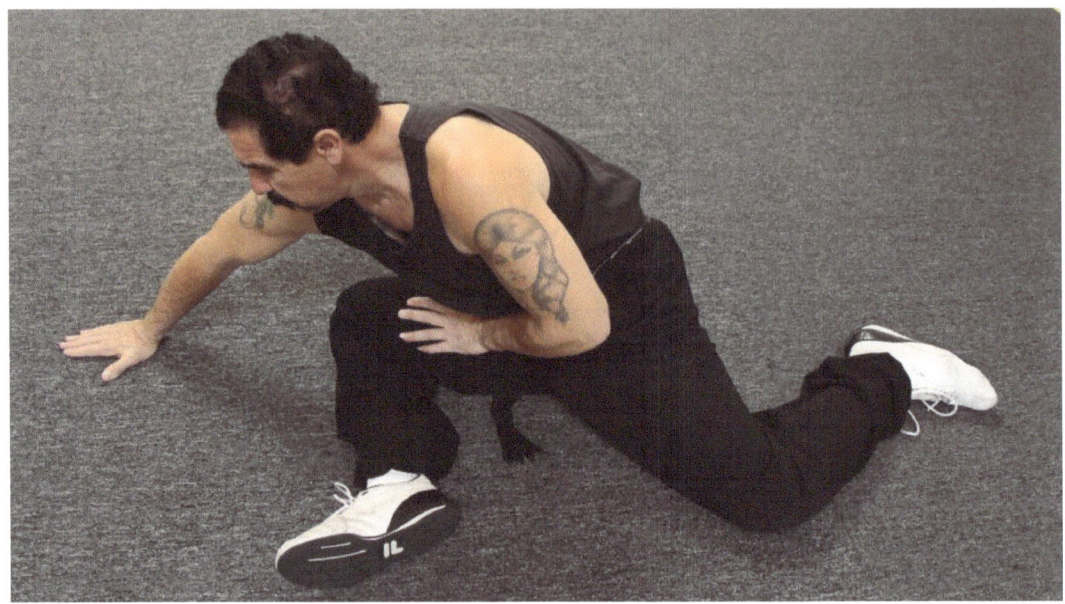

Position 3

- From position 2, inhale, and then, as you exhale, place the left hand even with the right hand, as if you were going to do a push-up.
- Relax breathing, and let muscles stretch.
- Bending elbows outward will increases the stretch.

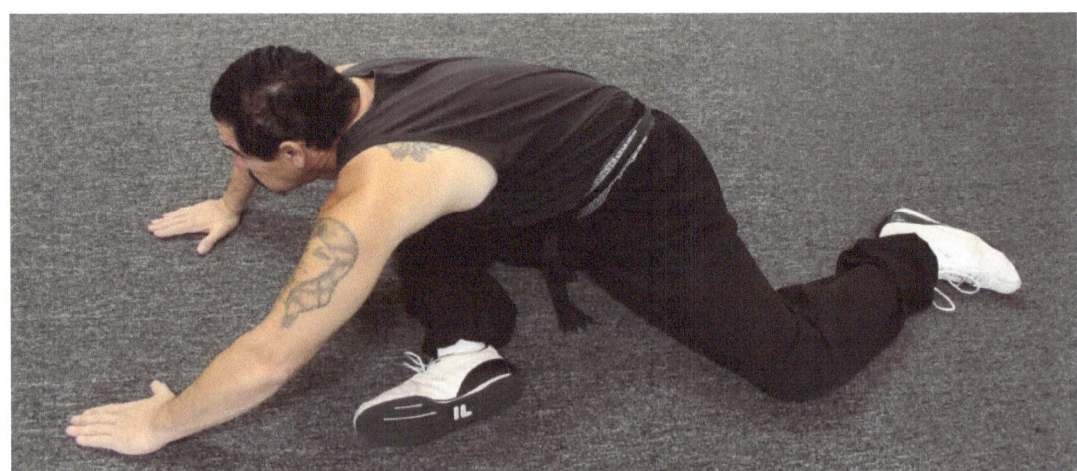

The objective with the hands is to be even and as far away from the body as comfortable. Tension in the leg indicates an uneven placement of hands. Relax breathing and let the muscles stretch.

Note: Maximize stretch by exhaling and bending elbows outward.

3-Part Angle Groin, Hamstring Stretch

Position 1
- Assume the seated position, and spread the legs as wide as possible.
- Place the hands on the floor, out in front as far as possible.
- Point the toes up and back, towards the knees
- Inhale and then as you exhale, pull with the palms as if trying to pull the chest to the hands.
- Repeat exercise through a couple of breathing cycles.

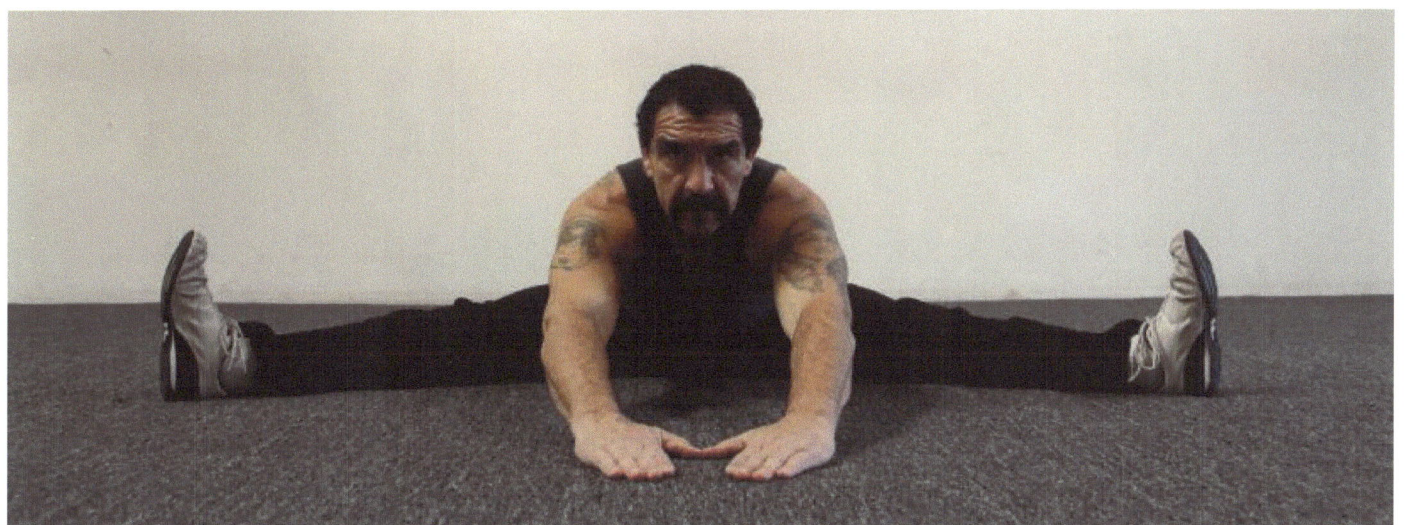

Assume the seated position, and spread the legs as wide as possible. The right leg will be at 2 o'clock and the left leg at 10 o'clock. Place the hands palms down, out in front of you as far as possible. Keep the toes pointed up and back towards the knees. Don't let the legs roll forward; that's a different stretch. Sink the palms into the floor. Inhale and then as you exhale, pull with the palms, as if trying to pull the chest to the hands. Once you get to that tense spot, relax the breathing and let the muscles stretch. Repeat exercise through a couple of breathing cycles.

Position 2
- Move both hands to the left, in between the left foot and 12 o'clock.
- Extend both hands out as far as possible.
- Inhale, and then, as you exhale, pull the chest towards the hands, again keeping the back straight.
- Repeat through a couple of breath cycles.

From the 12 o'clock position, move both hands out to the left, in between the left foot and 12 o'clock. Extend both hands straight out, get the palms dug in, inhale, and then, as you exhale, pull the top half towards the hands again while keeping the back straight. Proper form is with the back as straight and flat as possible.

Note: While exhaling, you are simultaneously lowering into the stretch position. Also, remember that proper form is the most important part of all stretches.

3-Part Angle Groin, Hamstring Stretch

Position 3
- Grab the left foot, or, if that's not possible, grab the outside and inside of the left ankle or calf area. Keep the toes pulled back and the back straight.
- Inhale and then as you exhale, pull the upper body toward the foot and extend the chin out towards the foot.
- Repeat through a couple of breathing cycles.

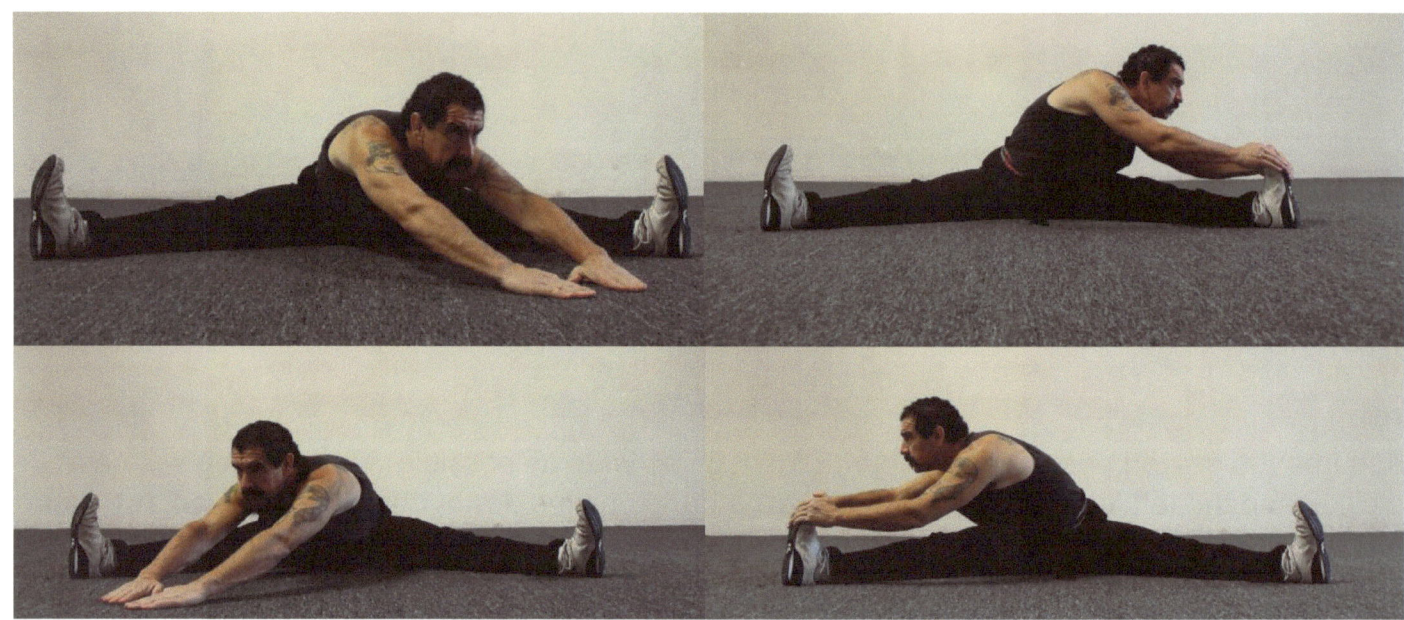

Repeat exercise positions 2 and 3 on the right side.

Relax; then take the hands all the way out to the left foot, and grab the left foot. If that is not possible, grab the outside and inside of the left ankle or calf area. Keep the toes pulled back and the back straight. Inhale, and then, as you exhale, pull the upper body toward the foot, and extend the chin out towards the foot. You should feel a stretch right around the back of the knee to the hamstring area. Repeat exercise positions 2 and 3 on the other side.

Calf / Hamstring Stretch

- Assume the seated position, with the legs extended out to 12 o'clock. Place the right foot on top of the left foot while pulling the left toes back.
- Grab the right foot at the toes, using both hands. If you can't reach far enough with the hands, use a towel.
- Inhale, and then, as you exhale, pull the chest out and down toward the hands, keeping the back straight.
- Repeat through a couple of breath cycles.
- Repeat exercise on other side.

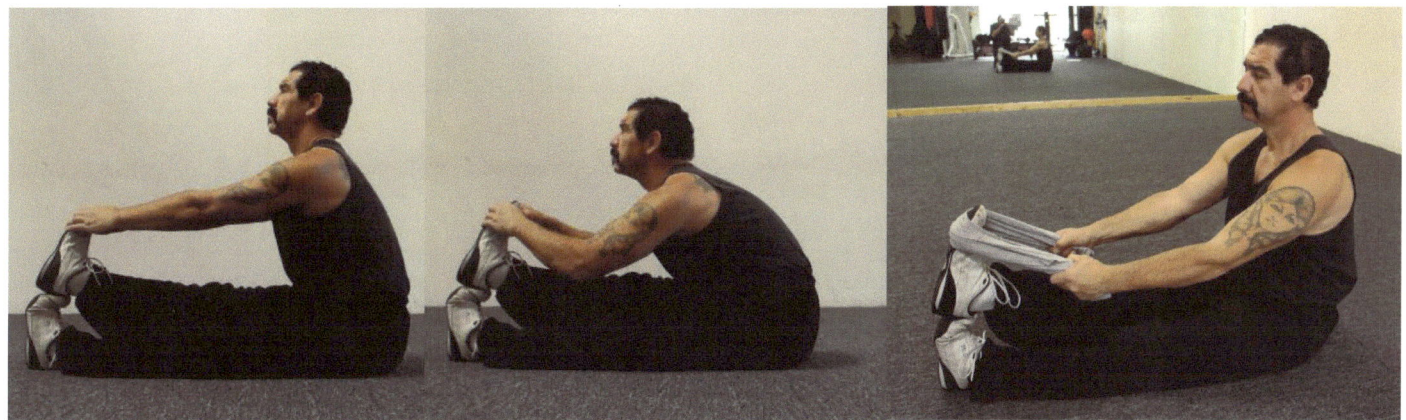

Assume the seated position, with the legs extended out in front. Place the right foot on top of the left foot, so it's automatically pulling the left toes back. Grab the right foot at the toes, with both hands. Tension on the bottom of the legs is a calf stretch, what I call a 'stacker.' If you can't reach the toes with the hands, use a towel. Wrap a towel around the back side of the toes of the top foot and utilize each end of the towel as a handle. Inhale and then as you exhale, pull arms back towards the body; move the chest out and down toward the hands, keeping the back straight, and attempt to touch the top toes with the chin. Repeat exercise on the other side.

Low Back Stretch

- Assume the seated position and cross the right leg over the left.
- Place the right arm behind you and place the left elbow over the outside part of the right knee.
- Inhale, and then, as you exhale, use the left elbow to twist and turn the body to the right.
- Repeat through a couple of breathing cycles.
- Repeat exercise on the other side.

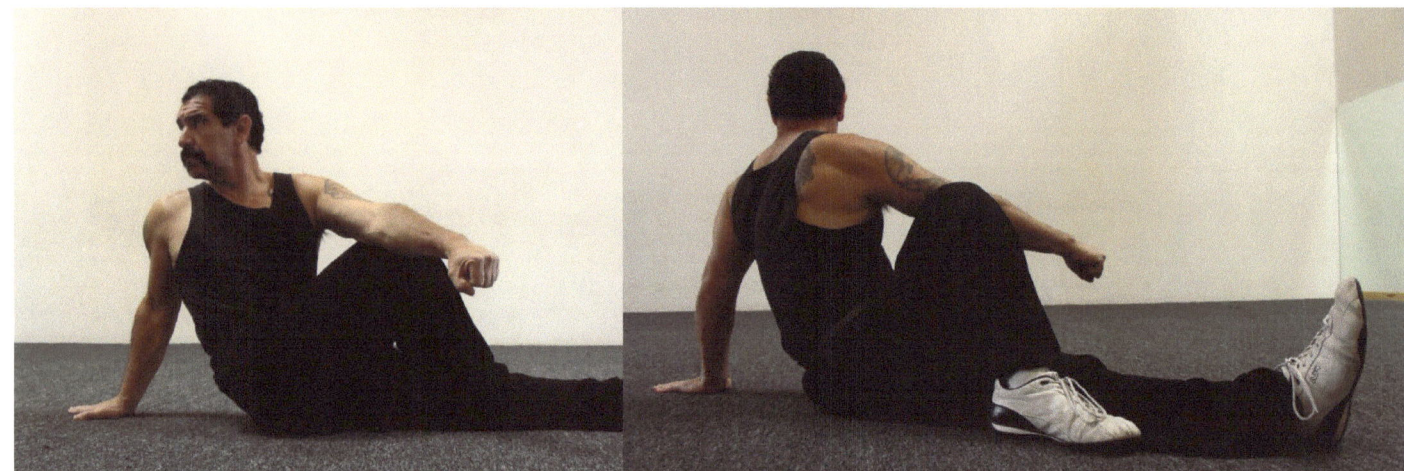

Assume the seated position with both legs out in front, and cross the right leg over the left. Place the right arm behind you and left elbow over the outside part of the right knee. Now, the elbow is going to be used to twist and turn the body to the right. The idea is to be able to twist and look behind you. Once the right elbow is straight, inhale, and then, as you exhale, twist to look backwards. Once the twisting look is in place, hold the position and relax the breathing. Repeat exercise on the other side.

Low Back / Glute Stretch

- Assume the sitting position, and cross the left ankle just past the right knee.
- Lay back like you're going to do a sit up.
- Place the left hand between the legs and the right hand on the outside of the right knee. Interlock the fingers, in the front of the right knee.
- Inhale, and then, as you exhale, pull the right knee toward the chest.
- Exhale, and then lift the chest toward the knee.
- Repeat through a couple of breathing cycles.
- Repeat exercise on the other side.

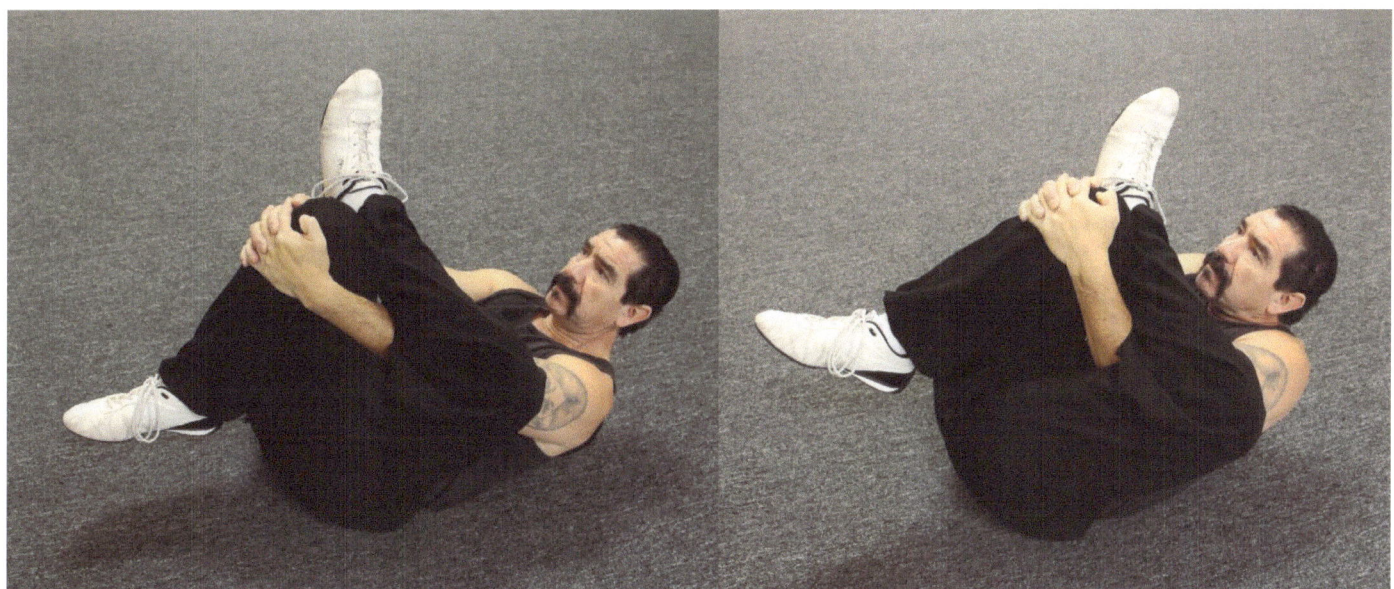

Assume the sit up position. Cross the left leg over the right leg and the left ankle just across the right knee. Lay back like you're going to do a sit up. Place the left hand between the legs, and place the right hand on the outside of the right knee. Interlock the fingers in the front of the right knee. At this point, you should feel a little stretch already. Inhale and then as you exhale, pull the right knee toward the chest, and lift the chest toward the knee. Hold the body in position, and relax breathing.

Note: If you can't reach the knee, use a towel. Wrap in front of right knee, and pull back with hands.

Assisted Neck Stretch

- Place left hand over the top of the head, and touch the right ear.
- Pull the head to the left, dropping the right shoulder down.
- Repeat exercise on the other side.

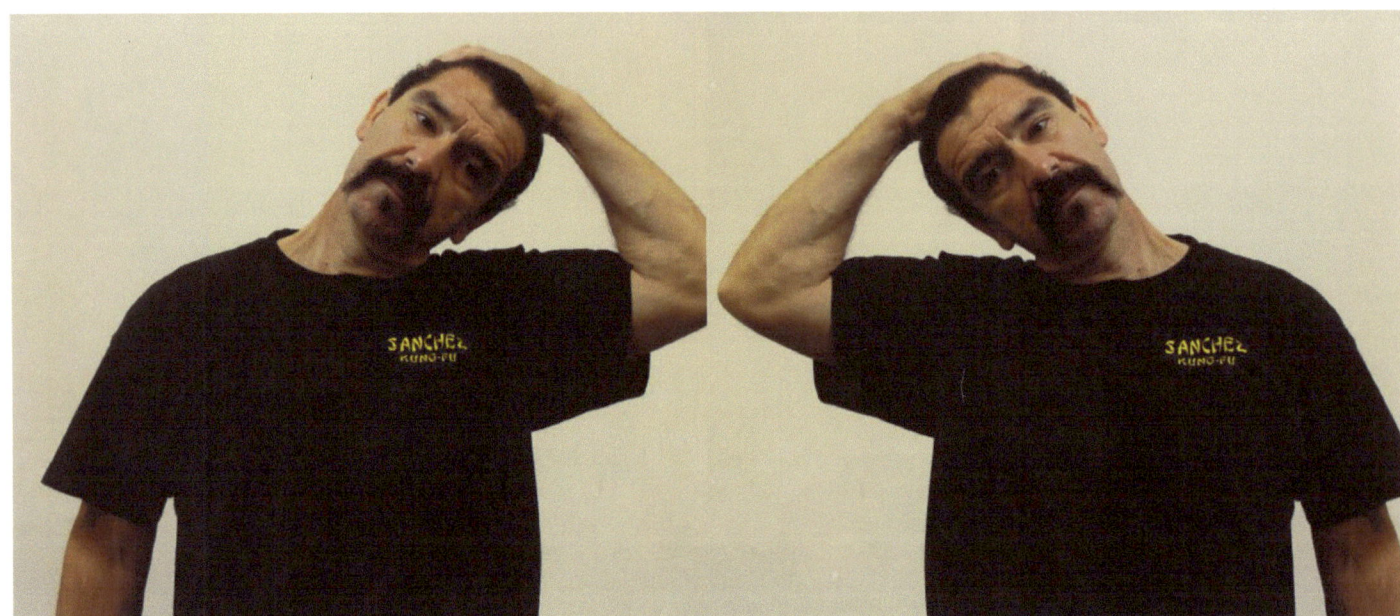

Assume the standing position, with arms at the side. Place the left hand over the top of the head, and touch the right ear. Then, pull the head to the left while dropping the right shoulder down. You should feel a stretch on the right side of the neck. Repeat exercise on the other side.

To get out of stretch, lift extended arm up over head to minimize straining.

Lat / Oblique Stretch

- Assume standing position, and spread the legs shoulders-width apart.
- Place right hand over the top of the head, and touch the left ear.
- Inhale, and bend the upper body toward the left foot.
- Exhale and feel the stretch on the right side of the body.
- Inhale deeply, and then, as you exhale, extend the right arm as far to the left as possible.
- Repeat exercise on the other side.

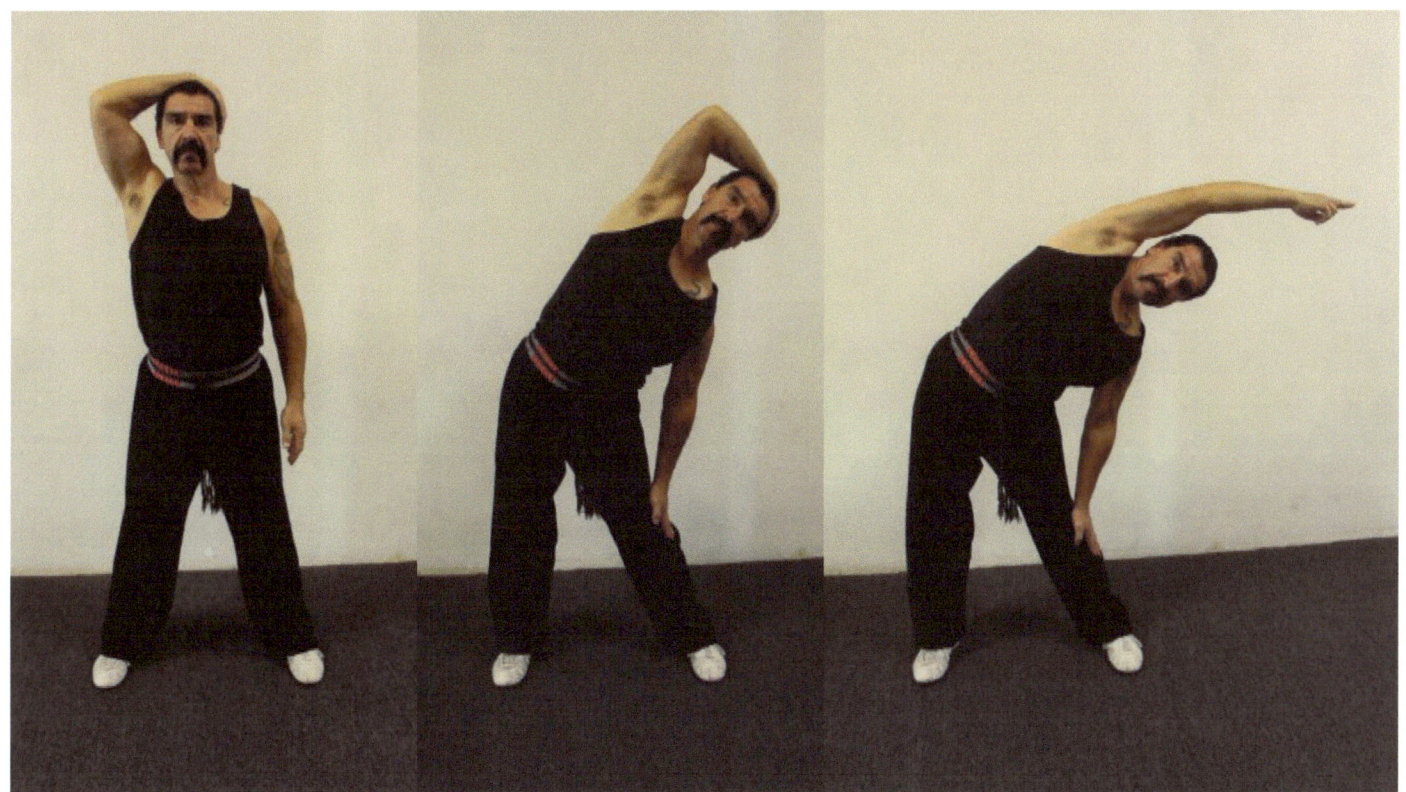

Assume the standing position. Spread the legs apart, to the width of shoulders. Start with both hands down at the sides. Place the right hand over the top of the head, and touch the left ear. Inhale, then bend the upper body toward the left foot. Relax breathing, and hold position for ten seconds; that's going to stretch the right side of the body. Take a deep breath in. As you exhale, release the left ear, extend the arm, and point the finger as far to the left as possible for an increased stretch. Repeat exercise on the other side.

To get out of stretch, lift extended arm up over head to minimize straining.

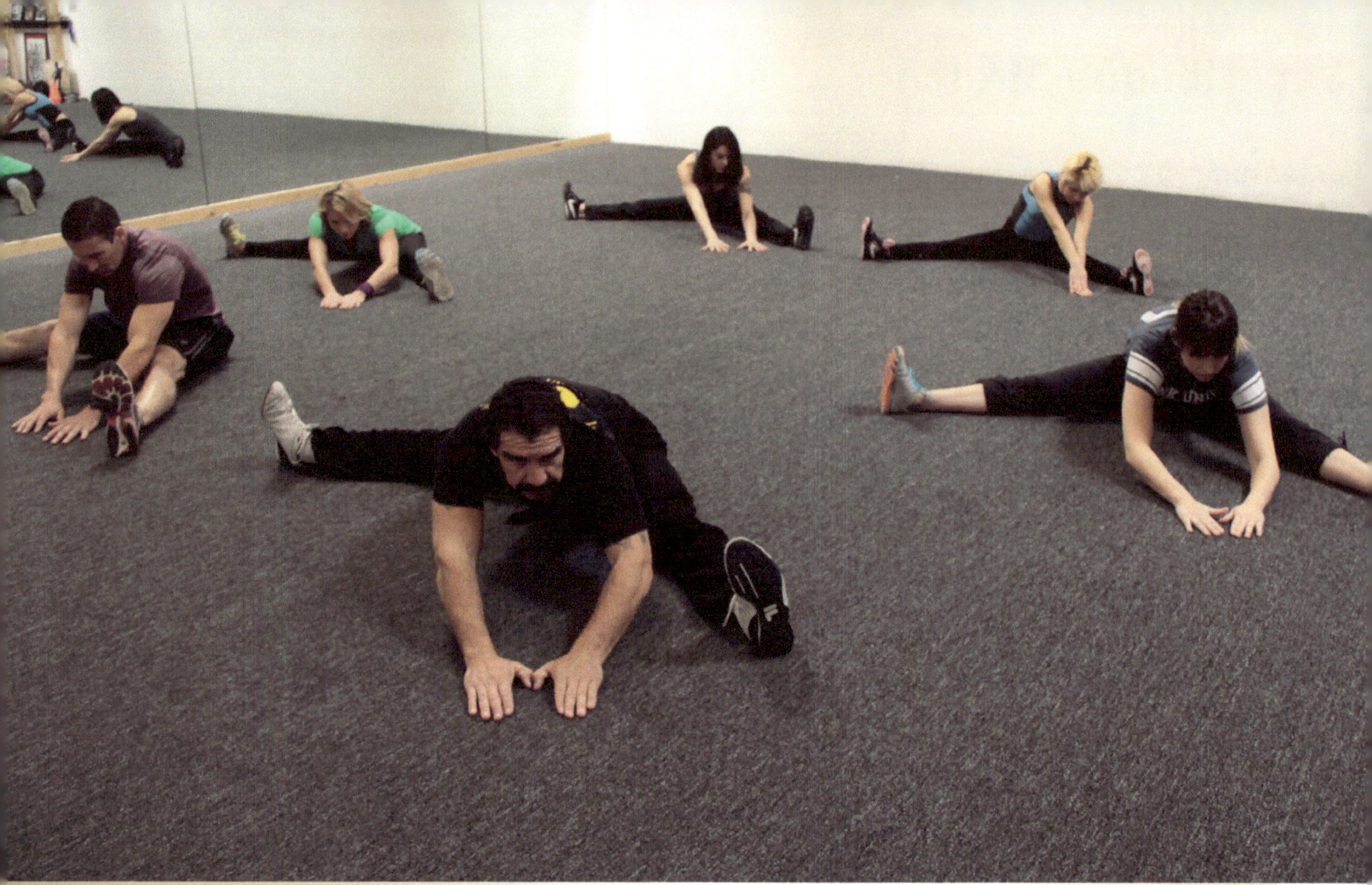

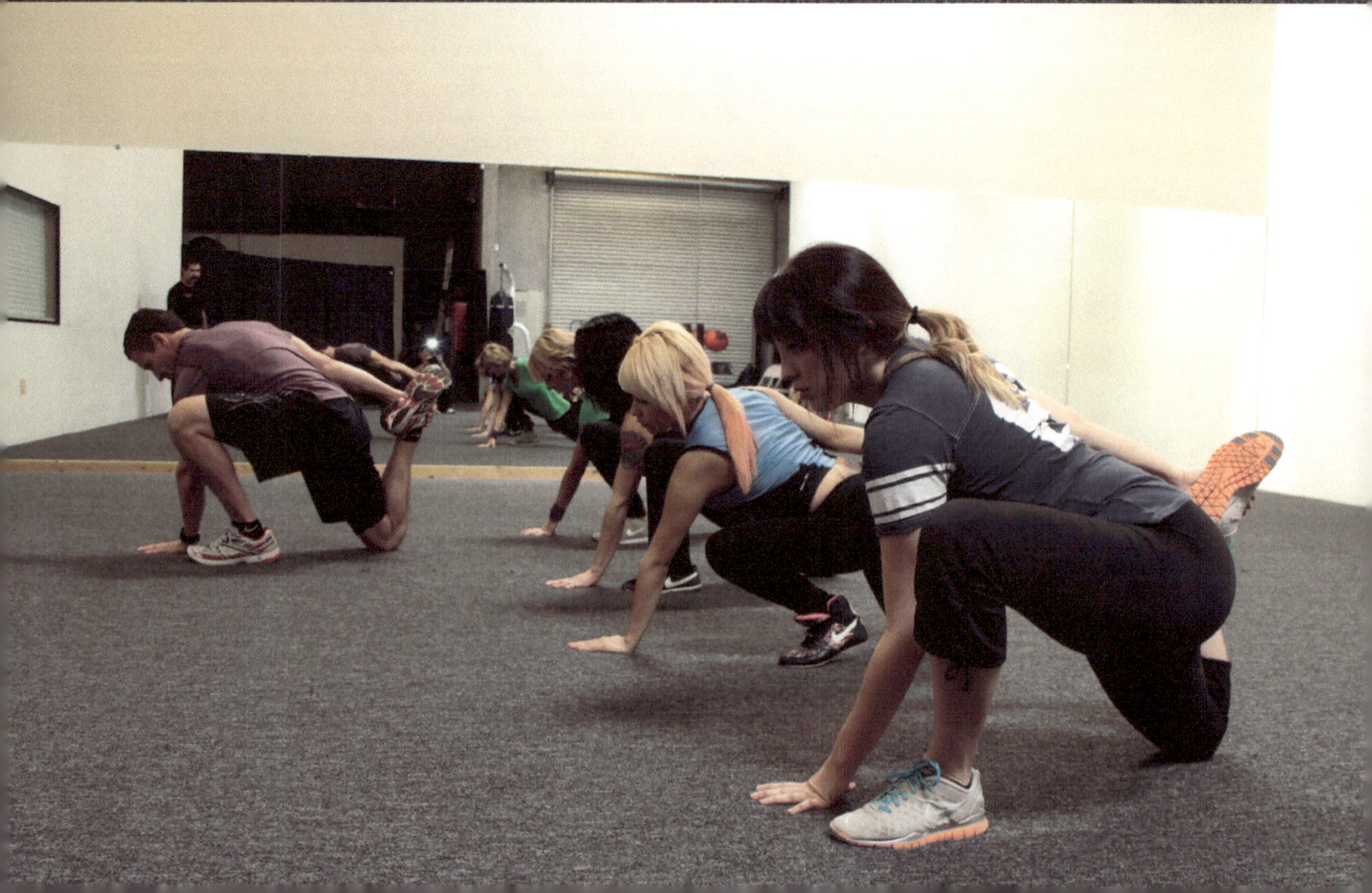

BIOGRAPHY

Sigung (Master) Manuel Sanchez

Born in Santa Paula CA.
36 Years Martial Arts experience
Sigung Manuel was introduced to his first martial arts moves at about the age of 10 by a family friend, deputy sheriff and Swat Team member Sgt. Juan Mendez, a technique he still remembers to this day. A few years later, Sigung Manuel began his formal training under the guidance of:

Great Grand Master Howard Lee: Founder and director of the Southern Shaolin Hang Ling Do Kung Fu Club.

Grand Master Eric Lee: Wun Hop Kuen Do/Kajukenbo. Undefeated forms and weapons champion. King of Kata.

Double Grand Master Ted Sotelo: Kajukenbo/Doce Pares Cacoy Canetes modified Corto Kurbada Escrima and Eskrido/Wrestling/Ground Fighting

Grand Master Keith Straughter: Kajukenbo/Aiki Ju Jitsu (technical & tactical)

Sigung Manuel is also a former weapons competition champion and was rated nationally in the top 10. He was featured in M.A. training magazine for his conditioning Push Ups, titled "Push Ups From Hell."

He has also been a bodyguard to many Executives, Celebrities, Families and Unmentionables. A financial recovery expert for Executives and Unmentionables: an expert in urban assault defenses, extreme self defense against 1 on 1 or multiple attackers, proficient in many traditional and non traditional weapons, actor, producer, movie stunt fighter with over 20 films to his credit.

Sigung Manuel was the first brown sash (belt) and youngest (age 17) to rank as bodyguard to Great Grandmaster Howard Lee, chosen by GG Master Lee himself. He is also the only student of G.G. Master Lee to be allowed to open his own school in the same town. He is the first of 5 worldwide to be promoted to Sigung (Master Rank) 8th degree black sash in the Southern Shaolin Hang Ling Do Kung Fu club.

G.G. Master Howard Lee realized that Sigung Manuel had a lot of anger and a unique fighting ability and a no fear attitude. This was partly due to the fact that at age 14 on a hog ranch his family owned he had to deal with castrating many large hogs, ride horses, bulls and steers and at a neighboring ranch as well as other reasons. By the age of 18, Sigung Manuel had accumulated more street fights than most do in their entire lifetime. G.G. Master Lee wanted to mentor and help channel that angry energy into a no nonsense method of self defense. The two spend many, many private hours doing so. At that time, Sigung Manuel's father even got him a bouncers' job by 18 at a friends' local rough bar to teach him a lesson and hopefully instilling some fear in him. It did not work. Sigung Manuel then began fighting these so called tough grown men and honing his skills. He would then share with G.G. Master Lee that a specific technique did not work as well as practiced. Instead of being disciplined by G.G. Master Lee, he was instead taught how to tighten up (perfect) his fighting skills.

Described in fighting terms as very explosive, Sigung Manuel's method of teaching training and conditioning is very unique and has many variables. But it all comes together to create and enhance your ability and agility for all angles of movement. Sigung Manuel tries not to bring too many hypotheticals to the training floor. He draws more from his real life experiences, confrontations and methods of applications for any given situation to defend your self successfully.

The teaching of forms and weapons Sigung Manuel learned from one of if not the worlds best, Grand Maser Eric Lee known worldwide as the King of Kata. An undefeated weapons and form champion with over 100 titles won, his teaching of explosive movements stop on a dime or continual flow are legendary. Sigung Manuel took that energy and knowledge in to competition favoring the 9 sectional whip chain as his weapon of choice, and won many championships.

Sigung Manuel's love, honor and respect to his Sifus are lifelong. Great Grand Maser Howard Lee is no longer with us, but Sigung Manuel carries on keeping a part of G.G. Master Howard Lee's legacy in every move. Rip Sifu

Pro level Students have included NFL players MLB Players, Pro Boxers, Law Enforcement Officers, Collection Agents, Body Guards and more.

Personal protection/Bodyguard clients have included Corporate Executives Officer (CEO's), Celebrities in entertainment, Pro Boxers, foreign counsel members, Kung Fu grandmaster and a group of unmentionables.

Among some of the many accomplishments Sigung Manuel is willing to share:

The first of only five worldwide to be promoted to 8th degree black belt
Sigung (Master Rank) Southern Shaolin Hang Ling Do Kung Fu
The first brown belt and youngest ever (17) to be bodyguard to Great Grand Master Howard Lee founder & director of Hang Ling Do
Internationally certified martial art teacher whkdia.com (MMA non sport)
Board member Wun Hop Kuen Do/Kajukenbo
Master council member Hang Ling Do Kung Fu Federation
Head master urban assault defense and extreme self defense and conditioning Southern Shaolin Hang Ling Do Kung Fu Federation
Advisory master of self defense techniques and applications Mountain Institute of Kung Fu and Tai Chi
Nationally rated weapons competition champion
Inducted 2013 Masters Martial Arts Hall of Fame

Inducted 2013 Martial Arts History Museum Honor Award
Member (SAG) Screen Actors Guild
Over 36 years martial arts experience
Proficient in many traditional and nontraditional weapons
Member of KOA – Kajukenbo-Ohana Association
Featured in MA Martial Arts Magazine

Sigung Manuel has a unique and wide range of technical and tactical methods/discipline of expertise of various martial arts.
Some of which include:

Southern Shaolin Hang Ling Do (5 animals) traditional/modified) 8th degree
Wun Hop Kuen Do/Kajukenbo (MMA non sport) 6th degree
Aiki Ju Jitsu (joint manipulation, proficient in pain compliance)
Chin Na (the art of seizing, locks and throws)
Chinese boxing
Hing Chong Li (joint destruction methods)
Grappling and ground fighting (non sport)
Urban assault prevention/explosive self defense
Stick and knife
Streets 101 and 102 (If you have to ask then it's not for you!)

Entertainment

Over 20 movies/stunt fighter/actor
Television, Asian fighting arts commercial lead fighter
Movie producer, Final Payback
Latin film group
Producer Hollywood stunt fight seminars with Art Camacho
Producer & Lead Urban assault prevention video with Grand Master Eric Lee, Sifu George Christie and Sifu Art Camacho

Motivational

Speaker – Teen Challenge
Speaker – Felons gang and clubs current & former members
Speaker – Security consultant to corporations & individuals
Creator - Fear No Mans Hands : www.facebook.com/FEARNOMANSHANDS

CURRICULUM VITAE

Logan T. Osland, D.C., C.C.S.P., C.S.C.S., Q.M.E.
4561 Market Street, Ste. C, Ventura, CA   93003
Phone (805) 644-4937 | Fax (805) 644-9038
loganosland@gmail.com | www.DrOsland.com

Education:
* Fresno City College, Graduated December 1990, Associate Arts Degree
* Cal-State University, Fresno August 1990 to May 1991
* Palmer College of Chiropractic West, Graduated December 1994,
Doctor of Chiropractic

Postgraduate Work:
* Associate Doctor, Wilson Chiropractic & Sports Medicine Clinic,
October 1994 to April 1997
* Owner Osland Chiropractic May 1997 to December 1997
* Partner, Wilson Chiropractic & Sports Medicine Clinic,
January 1998 to January 2004
* Owner Logan Osland Chiropractic, February 2004 to Present

Certification:
* State of California
   License to Practice Chiropractic, August 1995
   Radiography Supervisor and Operator, December 1995
   Qualified Medical Evaluator, April 2000
* Certified Chiropractic Sports Physician, March 1998
* Certified Strength & Conditioning Specialist, October 1998

Miscellaneous:
* President Elite Training 2002 to present
* President of the Ventura County District of the California Chiropractic,
   Association 1999 to 2001
* Saint Bonaventure High School Football Team Doctor 1997 to 2013
* Buena High School Doctor 2013 to present
* Foothill High School Team Doctor 2014 to present
* On- site doctor for local sporting events including:
   International Jet Sports Boating Association
   Adult Soccer Leagues
   Local Volleyball Tournaments

Memberships:
* California Chiropractic Association
* American Chiropractic Board of Sports Physicians
* National Strength and Conditioning Association

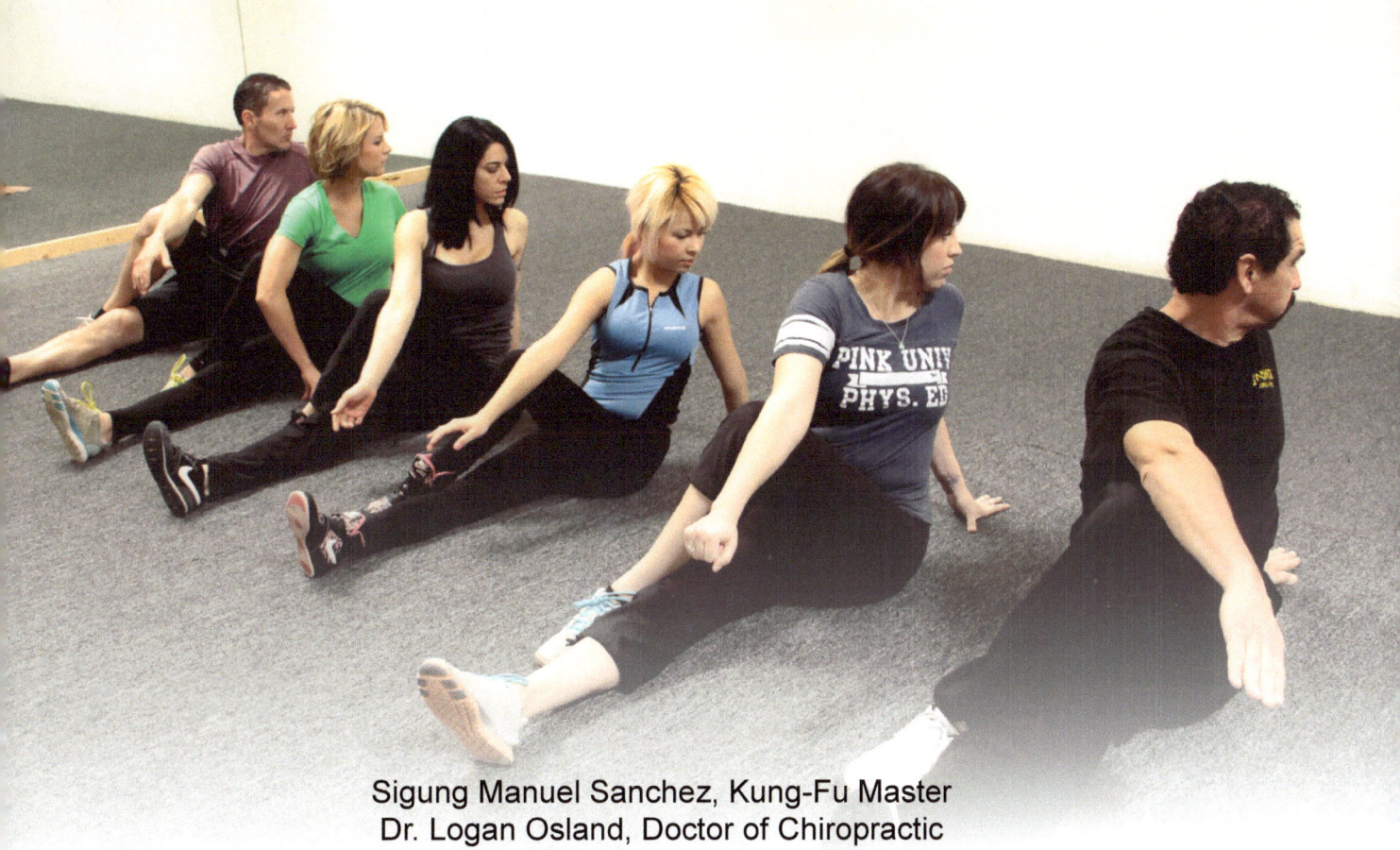

Sigung Manuel Sanchez, Kung-Fu Master
Dr. Logan Osland, Doctor of Chiropractic
Post Production= Sam Oldham
Photos= Dustin Gaeta A&D Photography
805-340-7655

Special thanks to
Sherrie Lemos, Krystal Kelly, Kasey Kelly &
Gennine Favazzo, Priscilla Quezada
Logan Osland Chiropractic
Chase Family
Bautista Medical Clinic
Mission Avocados
Sun Fresh Vegetables
Michael Morales C.L.S.W.
Wun Hop Kuen Do/ KajuKenbo
Southern Shaolin Hang-Ling-Do Federation
Sanchez Kung-Fu & MMA
Signung LLC
Turo LLC
AMJ Global LLC
Logo Screening by Rico Graphics
JulianneBlack.com
and
Dr. Art Malone Jr.

www.ingramcontent.com/pod-product-compliance
Lightning Source LLC
Chambersburg PA
CBHW041529280526
45792CB00004B/1435